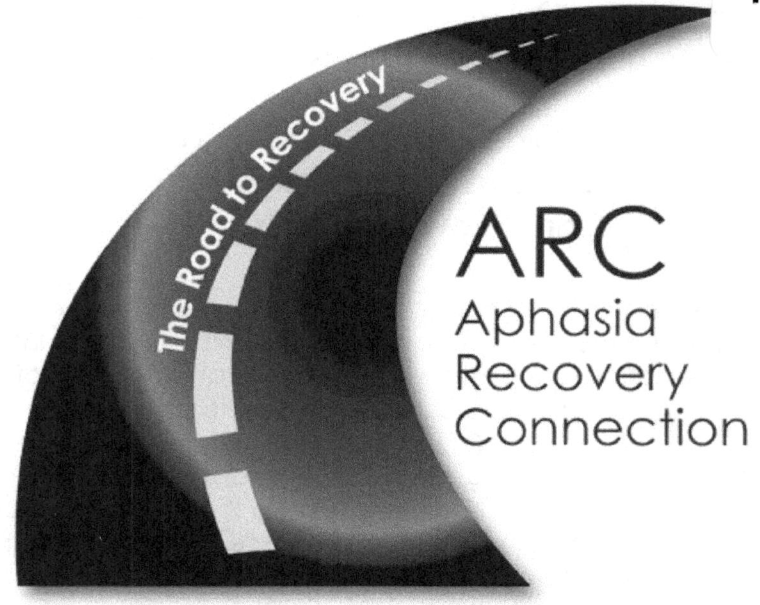

ARC'S

Guide to Living

with Aphasia

*Practical Advice
for People with Aphasia
& Their Loved Ones*

Carol Dow-Richards, ARC Director and
Amanda P. Anderson, MS, CCC-SLP

With David Dow

Aphasia Recovery Connection Mission

Our mission is to deliver compassionate support services to improve the quality of life for people recovering from aphasia and their families and friends.

We are committed to helping to end the isolation that aphasia brings.

We embody the values of collaboration, compassion, dignity, and acceptance.

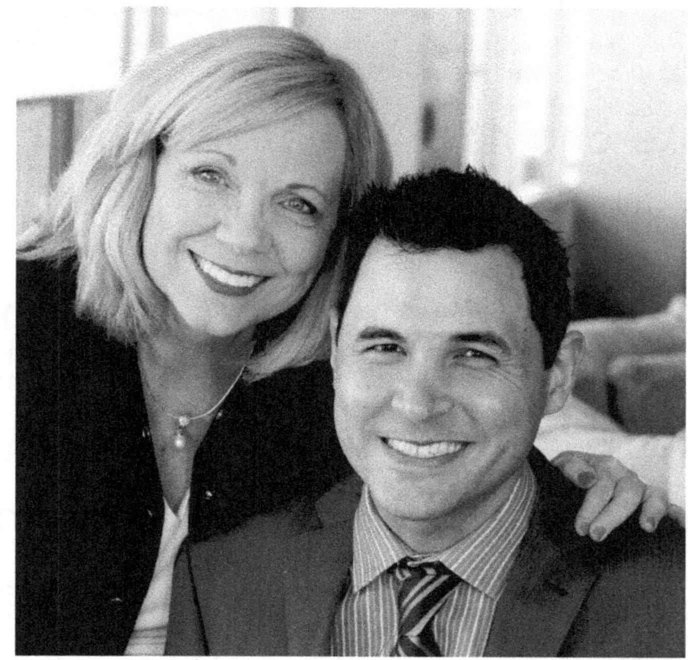

Photo: Carol Dow-Richards and David Dow

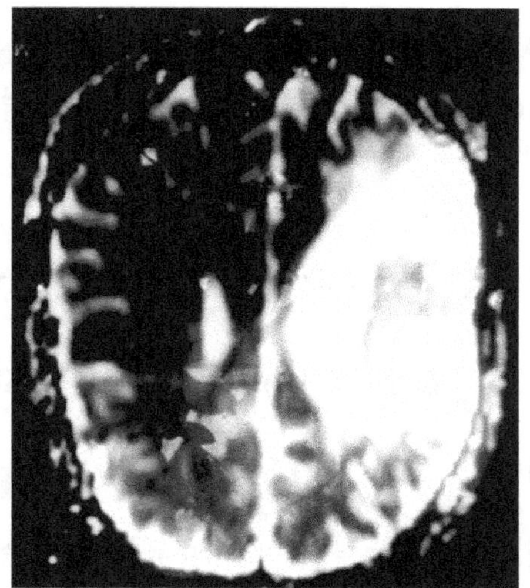

Photo: David's MRI from 1995. David suffered a massive stroke in 1995, resulting in aphasia and paralysis.

Progress: Slow and Steady

David Dow, Stroke Survivor

I had a stroke and have aphasia. I know how lonely the road to recovery can be. It is frightening, embarrassing at times, and overwhelming.

I hope this book will help you on your road to recovery. Recovery is often a long and slow process.

At times, it may feel like you aren't making any gains but gains come in many ways. Gains in speech, reading, writing, and processing and understanding language. Gains in confidence. Gains in motivation. Gains in understanding aphasia. Gains in adapting to an invisible disability.

You can start this book at any chapter. Share with family and friends because aphasia is a family issue. Communication is a two-way street, and with your new challenges, it is a good idea to enlist some help from others.

I hope you'll join us on ARC, our Facebook site, or face to face - on Virtual Connections video conference calls. Keep trying—it is a lot of work! I hope this book helps answers some of your questions. I encourage you to set goals and learn as much as you can. That is the best way to make progress. Day by day. Slow and steady.
You are not alone,

David Dow
ARC Founder

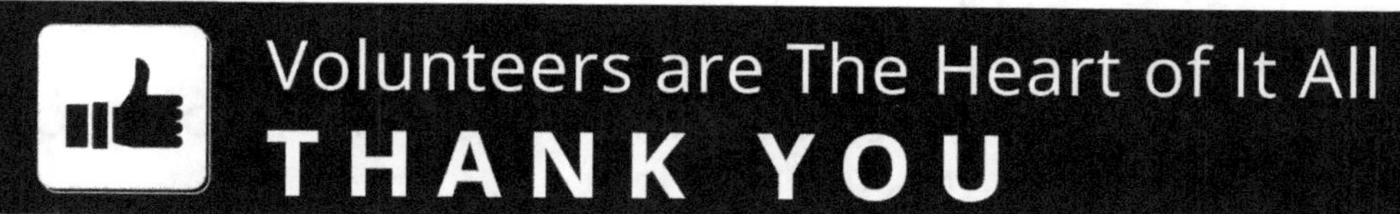

Carol Dow-Richards, ARC Director

I want to thank Speech Therapist and Co-Author Amanda Anderson for her dedication to this book. Her commitment to those with aphasia is heartfelt – and she has dedicated countless hours to bring this book to life as a volunteer for ARC.

We want to thank those with aphasia that shared their stories to bring the lessons from their journey. Their courage and determination have inspired others. Thank you to my son David, a stroke survivor and ARC Co-Founder – who first inspired Amanda and I to write this book.

Special thanks to our professional editor, Tamara Eaton, who has spent countless hours editing – but also has volunteered hundreds of hours for The Aphasia Recovery Connection getting to know real people with aphasia – which has helped make this book more aphasia-friendly by design.

And thank YOU! The purchase of this book helps support other families – like yours – that are navigating this challenging journey. You are not alone. We encourage you to join us on Facebook and get to meet other families face-to-face on Virtual Connections. I look forward to meeting you one day – virtually – online!

Carol Dow-Richards, Founding Director
Aphasia Recovery Connection, 501(c)3

Profits from the sale of this book support the mission of The Aphasia Recovery Connection.

About ARC

by
Carol and Jim C, Texas
ARC Members

"I've learned two big lessons since joining ARC. First, Everyone has a story. Everyone's story needs to be heard. They need to share it and we need to listen. The young professional who had a stroke and wasn't found for days. The mom who is struggling to raise her kids now that she has aphasia. The woman who had multiple strokes, but never gave up hope. All have stories.

"Second, We learned that we can help others, but also that sometimes we need help. Sometimes you are the mentor, other times you are the student. The ARC group enables us to both help and be helped. It is amazing how willingly members of this community share their thoughts with fellow survivors and friends.

"The ARC community is large and vibrant. It is a "community" in the true sense. It is an outlet for those with little language to communicate in a safe environment. Typos are ok. You don't need to write two paragraphs if two words will suffice. Both survivors and their care partners both have a voice."

Chapters
TABLE OF CONTENTS

Section/Chapter		**Page #**

INTRODUCTION

- ➤ **What Is ARC – Aphasia Recovery Connection?**
- ➤ **More About The Authors**
- ➤ **What Is This Guide?**
- ➤ **How Do I Use This Book?**
- ➤ **Disclaimer**

What is ARC?

What is Aphasia Recovery Connection?

Aphasia Recovery Connection (ARC) is an award-winning non-profit organization that works to help end the isolation for people recovering from aphasia. ARC was born from a personal journey of aphasia. Carol's son David had a massive stroke at the age of ten. There was little hope. He was paralyzed, unable to speak, read, or write. That was in 1995. Today, David has far surpassed anyone's expectations. He started ARC with his mom. He speaks at conferences and lives independently. But it wasn't an easy journey. ARC is the largest online Facebook Group for families dealing with aphasia with over 10,000 members. They also offer a Care Partner and Friends site as well as daily video conferencing options on Virtual Connections in collaboration with Lingraphica.

Want to learn more about ARC? Check out their website at: www.aphasiarecoveryconnection.org

More About the Authors

Carol Dow-Richards is an author, speaker, an award winning aphasia advocate and the Founding Director of the Aphasia Recovery Connection. After her son, David, had a stroke, Carol became a fierce advocate for people with aphasia. She facilitates support groups in Las Vegas and connects with families dealing with aphasia on a daily basis on social media and Zoom (video calls).

She's been a frequent speaker at national conferences and is featured on the American-Speech-Language-

Hearing Association's webinar, "Perspectives on Aphasia: Communication Breakdowns in Medical Settings."

Amanda P. Anderson is a Speech and Language Pathologist who specializes in aphasia therapy, both in-person and on tele-therapy. She is the author of the STAR Workbooks for Aphasia Rehabilitation. She is the recipient of the National Stroke Association's Raise Award for Outstanding Individual, and is a survivor of an internal carotid artery dissection, so understands the frustration of navigating care as a patient. She is the co-author of Carotid and Vertebral Artery Dissection: A Guide for Survivors and Their Loved Ones.

David Dow (Carol's son) suffered a massive stroke at age ten in 1995. He was hospitalized for three months due to a rare vascular defect called moyamoya. Since then, David has had 15 years of speech therapy with nearly 50 speech therapists. He met Amanda early on his recovery journey while she was a grad student working as his student clinician. Years later, they worked together again not as therapist and patient; but as authors. He's been featured in

People Magazine, *Good Morning America*, and *The Doctors.*

David's book, *Brain Attack: My Journey of Recovery from Stroke and Aphasia,* is an aphasia-friendly easy-reader available on Amazon. He co-authored *Healing The Broken Brain* with his brother, Dr. Mike Dow and Megan Sutton of Tactus Therapy. Both Dr. Mike and David were featured on an episode of The Doctors.

www.thedoctorstv.com/videos/how-dr-dow-s-brother-david-overcame-multiple-strokes

David is the inspiration for this book on living with aphasia. He offers continual support for people with aphasia through sharing his personal journey and challenges.

What is this Guide?

This book started with David's suggestion that people with aphasia needed a concierge. "Why do you say that David?" we asked.

David shared that the concierge in a hotel assists guests figure out what to do, where to go, and how to best budget their time and money while in a new city. David suggested people with aphasia need that same type of help. They need to know what the options are and how to best budget their time and resources.

> We need to help people like the hotel concierge, who helps people learn their options, costs, and what the best options are based on their own needs and budget. In a new city. In unfamiliar territory. People with aphasia need a road map. A concierge. To guide them."
> - David Dow

This book is designed to guide families on the road to recovery as they gain an understanding of aphasia, review rehab options, and find ways to boost their recovery potential. There are so many options that it becomes overwhelming for you to ponder different choices.

- Should you try an intensive aphasia program?
- Or something with social engagement?
- What about technology?
- Should you start with a tablet, such as the iPad?
- What apps are available?
- Should you utilize tele-therapy with an aphasia specialist via webcam?
- What does insurance cover?
- What does insurance NOT cover?
- Can you meet others with aphasia online or in person?
- Should you do therapy in a clinical setting?
- What activities are available?
- Are there workbooks or things you can do in my free time?
- What are some good strategies?
- How can my loved one be a better communication partner?
- How do you learn about aphasia research?
- How do you meet other families online?

This guide is intended to introduce the choices available. While some people can afford many options, others are left to wonder which one is best for those given more limited financial resources. They don't want to make a mistake on the journey, but are confused as to where they should spend their money. If they have little to no funds at all, they need to know how to maximize their insurance or perhaps find free or less expensive options. Sometimes they just need a good cry. Or to know they aren't alone. Or maybe they need someone to share this journey along the road to recovery.

While no two people with aphasia are alike, this guide offers you some options. Though we are not endorsing any particular method or idea, we are suggesting options to help you learn more so you can make smart choices along your own road to recovery.

How Do I Use This Book?

We understand that many people with aphasia may be unable to read this book, especially early on the aphasia journey. We hope that family members can read some portions of it to the person with aphasia when the patient is ready. Speech-Language Pathologists might also utilize parts of it for reading practice with their clients. If you purchased this for a Kindle device, you can have your Kindle or your Amazon Alexa read the book to you via VoiceView screen reader. More information is available on your kindle device or on Amazon's website.

Disclaimer

The information and advice provided here is not meant as medical advice in any way. The recommendations provided are for informational purposes only. We encourage readers to consult a medical professional before beginning any course of action based on the topics covered within this book.

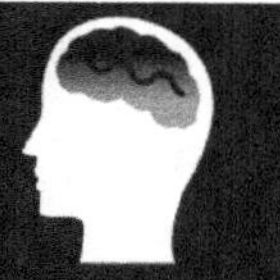

- ➢ **What is Aphasia?**
- ➢ **Does Aphasia Affect Intellect?**
- ➢ **What Causes Aphasia?**
- ➢ **What are the Most Common Types of Aphasia?**
- ➢ **What Does Aphasia Look and Sound Like?**
- ➢ **What are Other Speech Issues?**
- ➢ **What About Aphasia Recovery Timelines?**
- ➢ **Is There Hope for People with Aphasia?**

What is Aphasia?

Aphasia is a neurological disorder that results from damage to the language centers of the brain. Aphasia is an invisible yet devastating disability. People with aphasia may have difficulty with speaking (expressive language), understanding (receptive language), or both. Writing, reading, and math may also challenge people with aphasia. It is important to remember this: Aphasia is a language disorder and can mask a person's intelligence.[i]

While a person may appear impaired, especially in the beginning, this story may help you understand. Harvey Alter, former President of The National Aphasia Association shared this story at a conference Carol attended.

Land of Aphasia

Due to a stroke, Harvey's speech was slow and halting. Every day, before therapy, he stopped at a coffee shop. The owners had thick accents as they were from Portugal.

One day, they asked Harvey where he was from, as they did not recognize his accent. He replied, "I'm from Aphasia. It's a little country." They asked him to describe this country as they had never heard of Aphasia.

He shared that it's a place where mind and your mouth don't match. You are afraid to order in the restaurant. The telephone rings and you are afraid. The doorbells rings, you are afraid. You cannot tell the one you love how much you love them.

Once you are in the land of aphasia that is where you are. There are no planes to get out of Aphasia. There are no boats to take us away from Aphasia. You just wake up one morning and there you are in the country of Aphasia."

Does Aphasia Affect Intellect?

Often, people with aphasia are mistaken for being without intellect. However, they are indeed thinking and are still smart. But sometimes, others may not understand that their intellect is still intact since they have difficulty with language. That can be so frustrating. And indeed at first, you may have so many issues—you are overwhelmed by the changes. It can be confusing.

In the beginning, you may confuse left and right. Yes and no. Man and woman. (That often improves.) That is why many with aphasia need visual supports in the beginning such as a thumbs-up or thumbs down rather than a verbal yes/no.

David shares, "It is sort of like visiting another country where you do not understand the language. For example, if you go to Japan and do not speak Japanese, you will be confused when people talk to you. But you are thinking fine. When you go to write so you can communicate, you may discover you cannot write. When the person gives you something to read instead, you may find reading a challenge. It is terrifying to wake up and feel so disconnected to the communication happening around you."

What Causes Aphasia?

Aphasia is caused by damage to the language center of the brain. Aphasia can also result from other conditions that can cause a brain injury such as infection, head injury, aneurysm, dementia, or brain tumors.[ii]

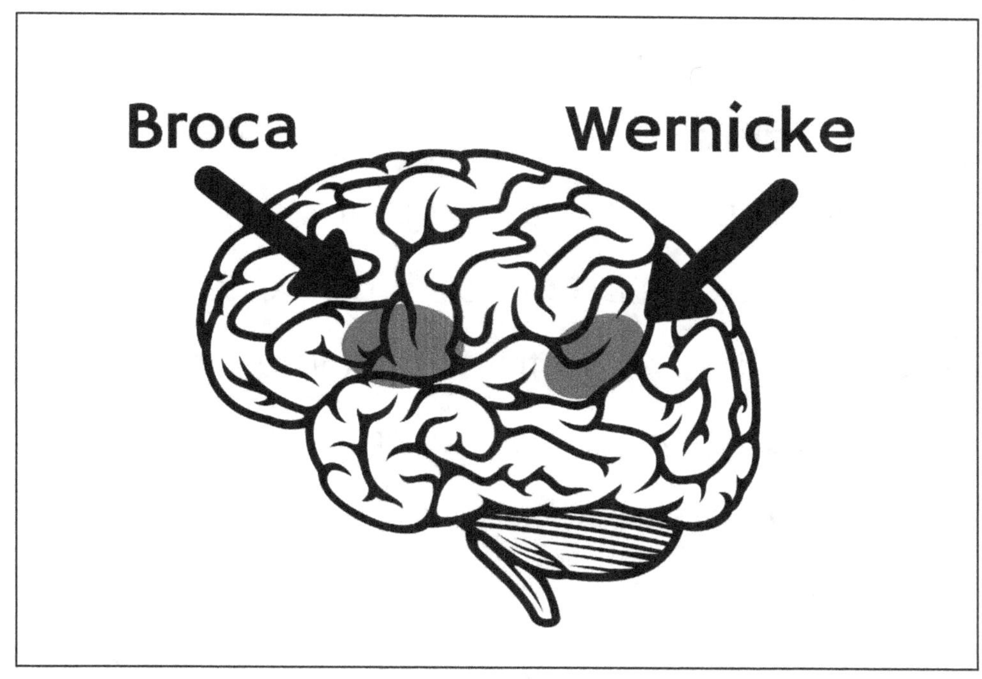

**Language Centers (Broca and Wernicke)
of the Left Side of the Brain**

Strokes

Strokes are the leading cause of aphasia. There are various types of strokes and no two are ever exactly the same and no recoveries are the same. It is important to know why you had a stroke to better understand both treatment options as well as to learn ways to reduce your risks of future strokes.

Ischemic strokes are caused by blood clots that obstruct blood flow to the brain and make up 87% of all stroke cases.[iii] When brain cells stop receiving blood rich in oxygen, even for a few minutes, the cells will die.

Ischemic strokes can be either thrombotic or embolic:

Thrombotic strokes result from a buildup of fatty tissue in arteries in the brain, sometimes where the artery has already begun to narrow. This blockage can stop adequate blood supply to language centers of the brain.

Embolic strokes are caused by clots in arteries that formed somewhere else in the body, such as the heart. Part of the clot can break off and travel to the brain, causing a blockage and an ischemic stroke.[iv]

Hemorrhagic *strokes* cause the remaining 13% of strokes.[v] This occurs when an artery inside the brain ruptures. The bleeding causes increased swelling and pressure in the brain resulting in damaged brain cells.[vi] Bleeding can be caused by aneurysm and arteriovenous malformation

(AVM). An arteriovenous malformation is "a cluster of abnormally formed blood vessels," which are vulnerable to breaking and bleeding. [vii] An aneurysm is a balloon-like pouch on an artery that weakens and can eventually burst.

Carotid and vertebral artery dissections are causes of stroke that are difficult to prevent. Trauma or underlying congenital weakness causes the layers of the carotid or vertebral artery to tear and bleed. The interior lining of the artery then bulges out which can cause blockage of blood flow to the brain.

Carotid and vertebral artery dissections are a leading cause of stroke in younger patients. Chiropractic neck adjustments, looking up for an extended period of time, roller coaster rides, car accidents, violent coughing spells, vomiting and even blowing up a balloon can cause dissections.

TBI

Another common cause of aphasia is a traumatic brain injury (TBI). This is sometimes from a gunshot wound, car accident, or other head trauma. These external forces on the skull and into the brain sometimes present added challenges, depending on the extent of the damage and area of the brain.

How Many People Have Aphasia?

Every year over 250,000 people in the United States are diagnosed with aphasia.[viii] Aphasia is more prevalent than Parkinson's Disease, Muscular Dystrophy, and Cerebral Palsy, yet most people have never heard of it.[ix] The National Aphasia Association found that 84.5% of people have never heard of "Aphasia."[x] Between 25% and 40% of stroke survivors have some form of aphasia.[xi] As of 2016, it was estimated that over 2,463,681 people in the United States were living with aphasia.[xii]

What are the Most Common Types of Aphasia?

A Speech-Language Pathologist will evaluate you to determine your type of aphasia. No two cases of aphasia are exactly alike. The part of your brain that was damaged is called a **lesion**. The lesion size and location will determine what type of language deficits you have. You might want to ask your doctor to look at your brain scans so you can see the area and have a better understanding of what happened.

You should not compare yourself to others you meet with aphasia because lesions vary greatly as do types of aphasia. Some people may be able to read, but not talk. Many people with aphasia can't talk, but some can write while others can't. For some, talking is easier but they may have difficulty understanding. Others will have all of the problems associated with aphasia. The good news is most people with aphasia will continue to recover and your aphasia will never be as bad as it was in the beginning. Below we describe the three most common types of aphasia. Your Speech-Language Pathologist will be able to evaluate you and provide a diagnosis regarding your exact deficits and more specific type of aphasia.

Receptive Aphasia

Aphasia can impact your receptive language. Wernicke's aphasia, fluent aphasia or receptive aphasia all refer to types of aphasia with comprehension trouble. Somebody with receptive aphasia may have difficulty understanding what others are saying. Sometimes they may need extra time to process spoken words in order to increase comprehension. In some cases, a person with aphasia may have no difficulty getting words out, but the words they use are incorrect and they often use made-up words. A person with this type of aphasia usually has difficulty recognizing that what they are saying is incorrect.

Carol recalls being in the ER with a support group member who had receptive aphasia. The doctor was drilling the patient quickly with yes or no answers, which the patient appeared to be answering. "Yes, No, No."

The doctor looked at Carol saying, "He seems to understand me just fine. I don't think you need to stay with him."

With that, Carol asked the patient, "Tom, do you have 3 children?"

"Yes," he replied. Confirming understanding is key to communication success for people with receptive aphasia.

Then, she held up her fingers, showing visuals. "Tom, do you have 3 children?"

He nodded.

Next, she held up her fingers, "Tom, do you have 2 boys and 2 girls?"

"No," he said, looking at her like she should already know that. But she wanted to show the doctor that this patient needed visual support and to confirm comprehension before dismissing her from the room after he had declared, "He understands just fine."

Communication access is a human right, especially in medical situations. Don't be shy to advocate on behalf of people with aphasia. Just like a person who needs a wheelchair should expect a ramp; a person with aphasia should expect communication support.

Expressive Aphasia

Expressive aphasia can range from severe, where the person may be unable to speak at all, to mild aphasia with occasional word finding difficulties, which is called **anomia**. Anomia is the sensation of having the word on the tip of your tongue but not quite being able to think of the word.

Expressive aphasia often limits a person's ability to participate in conversations, express basic needs and wants, and can be extremely isolating. The following are all different names for types of expressive aphasia: Non-fluent Aphasia, Broca's Aphasia, Transcortical Motor Aphasia,

Conduction Aphasia, and Anomic Aphasia.[xiii] They are all typically caused by damage to Broca's area of the brain.

Stroke survivor Lisa Wagner explained her experience when she first realized she had aphasia. She states, *"I think I talk right, but most people had no clue what I was saying.*

***Why would someone not tell me this? They were all so nice, nodding heads and smiling, so I thought I am fine...."* She wasn't fine. Aphasia had taken its toll.[1]**

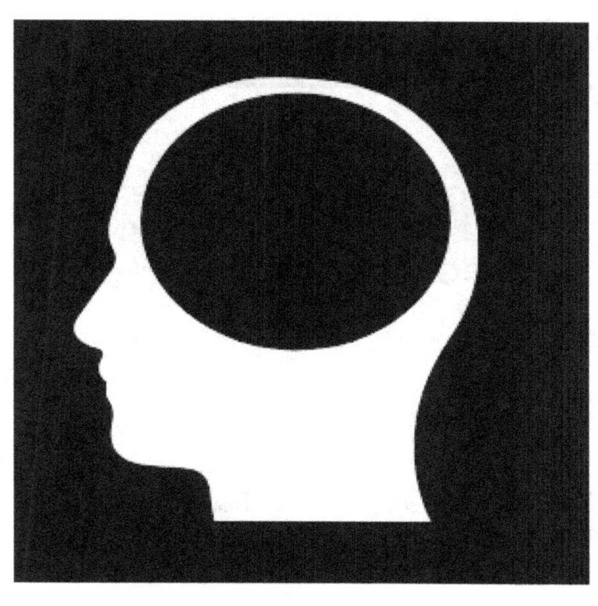

Global Aphasia

Global aphasia is the most severe type of aphasia because it combines both difficulty talking and understanding. Global aphasia is typical of somebody who has endured a severe stroke or brain injury that has damaged multiple areas of the brain.

> Carol recalls a time when she told David they had to hurry up and "hit the road." He stood there looking very confused. She repeated it, slowly and clearly, "We have to hit the road." David very carefully leaned his cane up against a car in the parking lot and literally bent down and "hit the road" as he touched the pavement. Now, she understood what the doctor meant when she said David had no abstract thought. David had taken her literally.

David was diagnosed with global aphasia. He had difficulty talking, understanding, reading, trouble with numbers, writing and even gesturing. With the help of SLPs and a lot of hard work, today he talks, understands, reads, and writes and is often an invited speaker to medical conferences today! People with aphasia can and do improve. It takes work. There is no magic pill.

David had both expressive and receptive aphasia in the beginning. Often, others would yell at him because they thought he could not hear. The real issue was he was having trouble understanding what was being said.

What Does Aphasia Look and Sound Like?

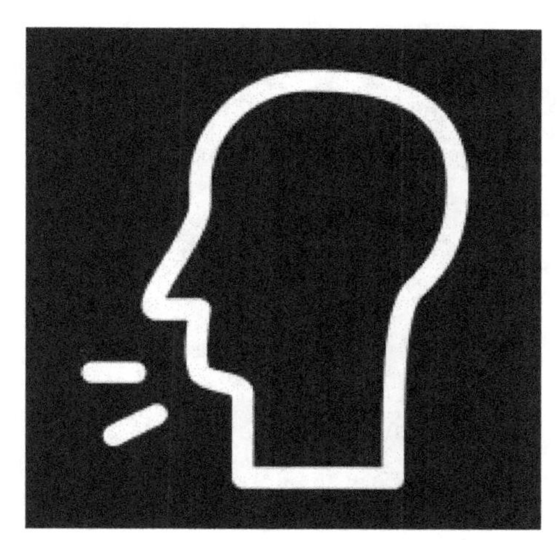

In the beginning it is important to know what you are able to do and what types of communication are difficult. Some people with aphasia can write what they want to say while others have just as much difficulty with writing as they do with speaking. If you are able to write, do it! Using communication in any form will be beneficial for your recovery.

Some people with aphasia can repeat words after they hear them, while others have difficulty with repetition.[xiv] If you are able to repeat after hearing a word or sentence, this is an excellent way to practice improving your expressive language function.

Aphasia presents itself in a variety of ways during attempts to communicate. Some of the frustrating symptoms of aphasia are listed in the table on the following page:

Symptoms of Aphasia

Acalculia	Loss of ability to complete mathematical calculations.
Anomia	Difficulty with word finding.
Circumlocutions	Talking around a word. Describing and using other words to explain what you are trying to say. This is actually a very positive technique and should be encouraged as a compensatory strategy.
Jargon	Fluent utterances that make little or no sense, often seen in receptive aphasia.[xv]
Perseveration	Getting stuck on a previous word and saying it over and over despite a new topic or question.
Phonemic Paraphasia	Substituting, adding, or rearranging the speech sounds in a word.
Semantic Paraphasia	Substituting an incorrect word for another with or without recognizing the mistake.

Other Speech Disorders: People with aphasia may also have other motor speech disorders, such as apraxia or dysarthria.

Apraxia	A disorder that impacts the brain's ability to control and coordinate muscles required for speech. Apraxia impacts motor planning function and can make it difficult to say the correct sounds in each word.
Dysarthria	A deficit that causes slurred speech secondary to oral and lingual (tongue) muscle weakness. Somebody with aphasia may present with difficulties in multiple areas or just one, depending on the size and location of the lesion caused by their brain injury.

Carol recalls David's first sentence was months after his stroke. "He suffered from both apraxia and dysarthria as well. She and David had gone thru a drive-thru window and she handed him his food. "Ank ou om," he said. She recalls being thrilled to hear his first three-word sentence, "Thank you mom." Progress was slow, but it was indeed progress. Many, like David, may have aphasia as well as other language challenges. With time, these tend to improve.

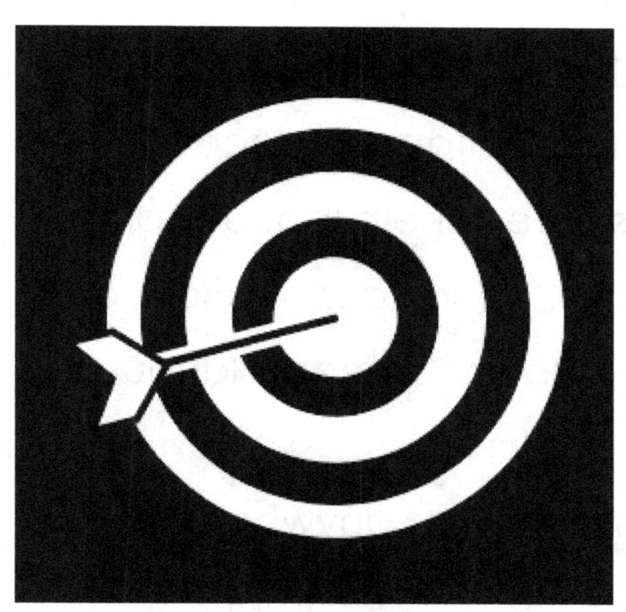

What About Recovery Timelines?

Just as the severity and type of aphasia vary from person to person, so will your recovery. Many factors determine how well someone with aphasia will be able to recover including: the size and location of the brain lesion, family support, age, motivation, amount of social interaction, activity level, and access to therapy.

There is often some spontaneous recovery that occurs within the first few hours and days after a stroke or brain injury. This is a result of the reduction of swelling in the brain, neuroplasticity, and overall restoration of tissue function in the brain.[xvi] As your body recovers in the first few days, people may see a dramatic increase in speech and language function. Also changes in metabolism and reduction of abnormalities of blood flow caused by the stroke or brain injury help promote spontaneous recovery.[xvii]

The next few weeks are considered the subacute phase where the brain begins to form new neural connections and begins neural reorganization to help speech and language recovery.[xviii]

The chronic phase of recovery can last anywhere from a few months to years and even decades.[xix] Improvement varies from person to person but recovery has been noted to occur long after the initial stroke or brain injury. The National Aphasia Association states that recovery from aphasia can occur over a period of years or even decades.[xx] David's most dramatic gains came nearly six years after his stroke.

Many members of Aphasia Recovery Connection have also shared that they have experienced continued gains many years after their diagnosis of aphasia. Connie Snell remarks on her husband's continued progress with speech therapy and says, "It will be two years since my husband's stroke. He has been in Speech Therapy the entire time and we are still seeing notable improvement."

And, remember that the goal is communication success. While talking may be the goal, there are many strategies to learn to support your aphasia challenges. We believe that you should focus on getting better and utilizing strategies and tools over the next weeks and months so you can communicate.

Remember, communication is not just about talking. It can be a hug, a gesture. It can be pointing to a picture. It can be using a device to give you support and peace of mind.

What Hope is There?

Although aphasia is indeed a very complex and difficult language disability, there is hope. Over the last decade there has been lots of research on the brain's ability to repair itself. But the will, determination, and resilience are qualities that you need to optimize your recovery. It is important you maintain a belief in yourself and keep working at it without giving up! It is common for survivors to at times – want to give up. Take some time to adjust and cope – and then get back to work!

There is no "right" or "wrong" way to cope as it is your own journey. It is sometimes tempting to compare yourself to other people who have had strokes, but it's best to keep in mind that your stroke and your recovery is unique to YOU!

Meeting others with aphasia is often very helpful as you connect with others that have been on this same journey.

We invite you to join us on the Aphasia Recovery Connection Facebook group site. You will meet others, be able to learn and share your experiences, ask questions, and most of all you'll find a group who is hopeful, positive, and caring. There, you can learn, share, and connect.

Self Evaluation:

➢ **What kind of stroke or brain event did I have? Or what caused my aphasia?**

____

➢ **Can I talk?**

____

➢ **Do other people understand me?**

____

➢ **Do I understand what people tell me?**

____

➢ **Can I write?**

____

➢ **Can I read?**

____

➢ **Can I do math problems?**

____

➤ **Do I need visual support to understand others?**

____

➤ **What are my goals for improvement?**

____

➤ **What are my best strategies to communicate?**

____

Other Notes:

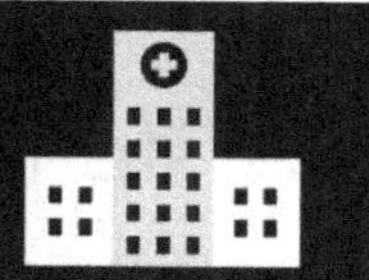

- What Happens (Or Happened) In The Hospital?
- What Tools Can I Use To Communicate With Nurses And Doctors?
- What Are Helpful Things To Let Nurses And Doctors Know?
- What If I Have Problems Swallowing?
- Who Are All These People? Your Recovery Team?
- What Should Visitors Know About Me And Aphasia?

Aphasia: In the Hospital

What Happens (or happened) in the Hospital?

Hospital stays vary widely depending on the severity of the stroke or brain injury and what type of medical care is needed. A person who has had a stroke typically spends an average of six days in the hospital.[xxi] Patients who are stable may start to receive rehabilitation therapy as soon as two days after their stroke.[xxii]

The initial shock of realizing you are unable to communicate is terrifying and devastating. Your body is still recovering from the injury to your brain, and you might not be able to figure out how to reach out to nursing staff or family. Honestly, they may not be sure how to best communicate with you, either. Not all nursing staff have received training to understand aphasia.

Carol recalls being in the ICU with her son David: "I really believed we would be home soon and he would be fine. He *had* to be fine. My brain could not even imagine that his disabilities would be with him for life. I think that was my way of coping. Often denial becomes a way to cope. But eventually, we had to realize that his aphasia was not going away any time soon. Nor was his paralysis. And we had a very long road ahead of us."

"While I believed we would be home soon – his hospital stay was nearly three months. During that time, I never left the hospital and slept in his room. With him being only ten and unable to communicated, it was imperative that I stay".

What happens during the time you are in the hospital is going to be unique to you, the cause of your aphasia, and the protocols at the hospital you are in.

Remember, do not compare yourself to other people.

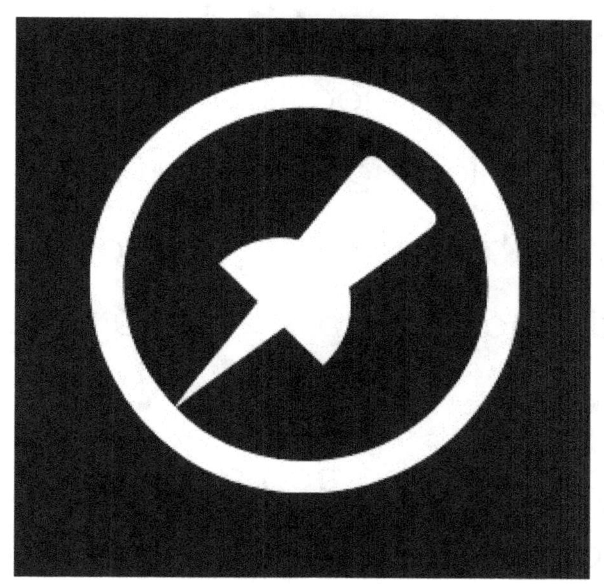

Your case is uniquely yours. If it is a small stroke, you may even be discharged within a day or two. Remember, every case is different. What people with aphasia do have in common is this: they need patience and lots of it! They need staff with an understanding of aphasia and they need to know how to communicate with them. Patients need tools to help them communicate, but our polling shows that the majority of families feel they are not given enough support or resources – if any.

Aphasia Tip

What Tools Can I Use to Talk to Doctors and Nurses?

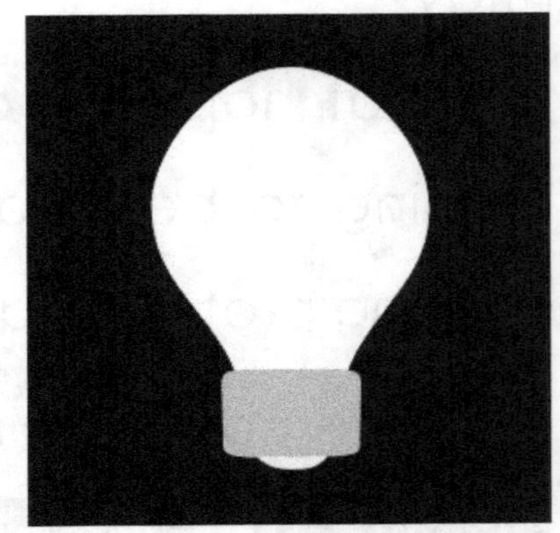

ARC members often share the lack of aphasia awareness and communication strategies within the hospital itself, which leads patients to feel even more vulnerable. On the following page is a basic communication board that may be helpful to you as it offers visuals. You can have somebody make a copy so you can point to the pictures.

Ask for a clipboard so you can keep the communication board with you. There are also communication board apps for your smartphone—some are even free. To find them, use the search terms "communication board aphasia." There are versions for both smartphones and tablets. One of our favorites is the Tactus White Board that can be found at https://tactustherapy.com/app/alphatopics-aac/.

The Lingraphica App, Small Talk-Intensive Care (Found here: https://www.aphasia.com/smalltalk-aphasia-apps/) is helpful for hospital use to show medical needs with pictures.

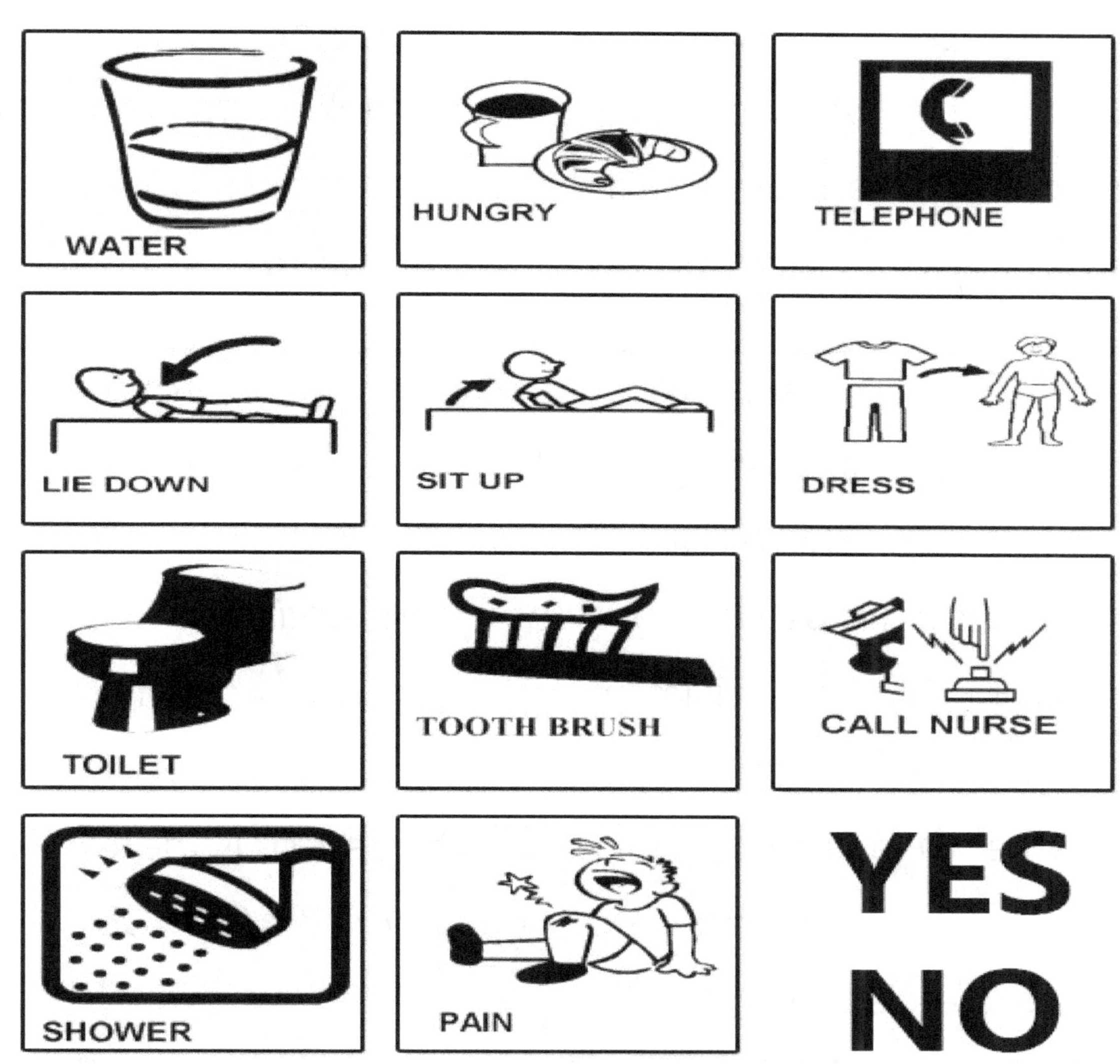

Basic Communication Board Example

Remember, no two people are alike. Your Speech Therapist may offer a different communication board for you. Some use words, some use pictures. And – in the first few days – some people are unable to use communication boards at all.

Some people leave the hospital without an understanding of aphasia. They are looking for resources. Many aren't even sure what it is called or even how to spell aphasia to begin their search for information.

> Carol shares, "When David had his stroke, we found ourselves very frustrated and afraid, terrified really. Initially the doctors didn't explain aphasia to us as they were concentrating on saving his life and limiting the damage from the stroke. As he lay in bed unable to speak, read, write, or even understand, I wondered, *Is there any hope? Is aphasia permanent? How do people deal with this?*"

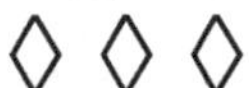

ARC member Lisa describes her frustrating experience in the hospital:

"Tankfew." I said.

My nurse responded to me with, "What?"

Sigh. "Blysiy tankfew." My hand reach my chest and pat my heart.

My husband added, "She's saying thank you."

"Oh you're welcome, hon," my nurse replied on her way out the door. I think, *"My name is not hon. My name is Lisa. Can't she read the stupid sign on the door? Why can't I talk? What happened to me? Why am I lying in bed and not home? John is here with me. What the hell is going on?"*

Later my nurse returned, "Time to draw more blood, hon. How are WE today?

I think, *"How are we? Really?? Let's see, I am not able to talk, the doctor keeps saying I have a stroke and it might take time to talk again, IF at all.*

So WE are scared to tears, can't do anything and stuck in bed with YELLOW socks on and not allowed up. That's how WE are today. But in fact I just try to be calm and let her draw my blood and leave.

As the nurse leave I say to her, "Ru nraw dreff. Nraw del tru mwaaa.

"What?"

Sigh. I meant to say, "I'm not deaf. Do not yell at me. And leave me alone."

My husband said, "She said thank you."

Another ARC member shared that he pressed the nurse's button and heard the response, "Can I help you?" *Silence—he could not talk. He pressed it again. Silence. He tried again and again.*

Finally a nurse came to his room and he was met with anger and frustration. "Do NOT press the button again and again. TALK into the microphone." She demonstrated it and stormed out of his room.

He could NOT talk. He did have needs. Important needs. Human needs. He wet himself. Left to feel humiliated and disgraced, misunderstood and vulnerable, he cried. He was the one who was angry and frustrated! How could a nursing staff not know that he could not speak?

ARC member Charade describes how she discovered she was having trouble with her receptive and expressive language: She explains, "Well, I thought that I spoke fine after my stroke. I thought that my family, my doctors, nurses and physical therapist, occupational therapist and my best friends were talking different tongues, like a Punk TV show. I didn't want a speech therapist. I studied AP English and AP history. I thought my right side was disabled not my speech. I did not realize at first my talking was not intelligible to other people.

"After 2 weeks, when my father visited me, I decided to tell everyone there, hey speak English please I was bothered about the different language.

I spoke English and Spanish fluently, I read Spanish and English, and write well. So I told my father about that, and he didn't understand. He looked sad, and he wrote you have aphasia.

I was puzzled, he explained speech disorder, and he said my speech is mumbles and everyone couldn't understand my speech. I was ashamed. I was very confused, and I cried and I will not speak anymore. However I read, my dream world."

Charade, like many patients, struggled to understand what had happened to her speech. The paralysis was visible. Aphasia is invisible.

Sometimes patients may not recall being told they have aphasia. Some are not told or if they are it may be so brief a mention that they are unsure how to spell it to research at home. It is indeed a very overwhelming time for both the patient and their family.

ARC member Thomas shares his story: I never knew about aphasia until about a year ago when I saw a video with a young lady that talks like me. I didn't know there is a word for that! It had been 14 years and there is a word for that!?!

I really gave my doctor heck when I saw her the next time. She apologized and said that it is only a part of the problems that I have from my head injury and she didn't know it would mean that much to me. Then, she started telling me about different forms of aphasia and I got confused again!

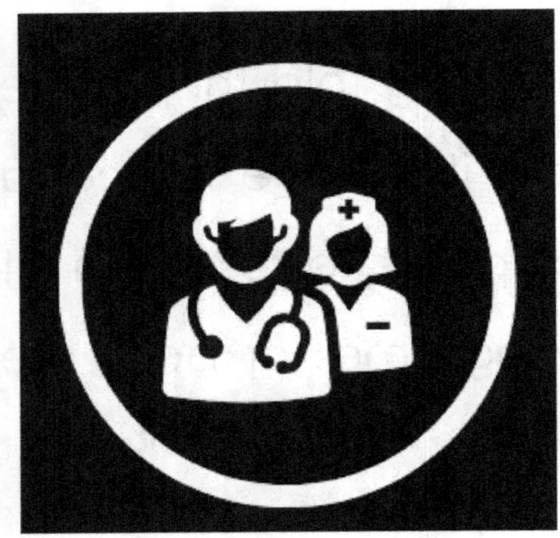

Even medical workers have difficulty understanding the needs of somebody with aphasia.

Carol recalls visiting an ARC member with aphasia on one of her travels. Suddenly he was unable to use his right leg and the left side of his face drooped. They rushed to the ER knowing these were classic stroke symptoms.

In the ER, the doctor started rattling off information very quickly so Carol said, "He has aphasia." The doctor continued on at the same speed, seemingly ignoring her or perhaps not knowing how to adapt his communication style for a patient with aphasia. Next, a technician came in and the scene was repeated, and then again with a nurse. She went to the nurses' station and asked for a piece of paper, clipboard, and pen.

She wrote this down for him:

- **I have aphasia.**

- **I worked as an engineer.**

- **Aphasia does not affect my intellect.**

- **Please reduce your rate of speech.**

- **Emphasize key words.**

- **I can read. Write down key words.**

- **I communicate with a whiteboard app on my iPad.**

Each time Carol and David visited him over the next week, he proudly showed the clipboard he kept in bed with him and he would give us a high five. Upon discharge, he sent us a photo of himself holding up the clipboard, pointing to it with a thumbs-up. He was so thankful to have this simple reference to show the staff. It empowered him to self-advocate and enhanced his communication with staff and visitors alike.

You might ask a loved one to adapt this example for your own use during your hospital stay. If you are not in the hospital as you read this, you can still make a communication list and keep it handy. This way, if you ever return to an ER or when you visit a doctor's office, you are able to self-advocate for your own needs by sharing information. It is remarkable what a few pieces of information about aphasia can do to improve communication and help others help you. In **Appendix A**, you'll find a template to complete with your own information.

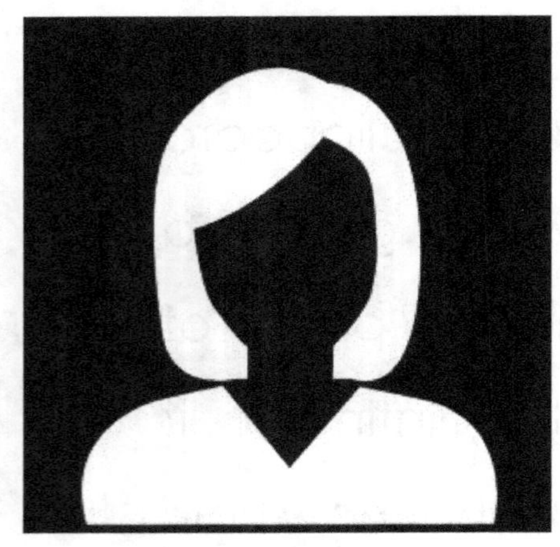

Ask your Speech Therapist

> ➤ *Please help me make a list to tell my medical people about me.*

> ***You could also add other information you want others to know such as:***

- family
- phone number
- names of your family
- a photo.
- Ways to help the hospital staff better serve you.

The first few days with aphasia are naturally confusing, scary, and exhausting. You may feel trapped and frustrated because of your inability to communicate. We have provided questions in bold print you can point to and use to communicate with nursing staff and caregivers.

Try your best to use any modality of communication that is available to you. Nod "yes" and shake your head "no". Point, make facial expressions, and use any words you can even if it isn't the exact word you want. Some people struggle with yes and no in the beginning. Using a thumbs-up or thumbs down adds a visual that may help understanding.

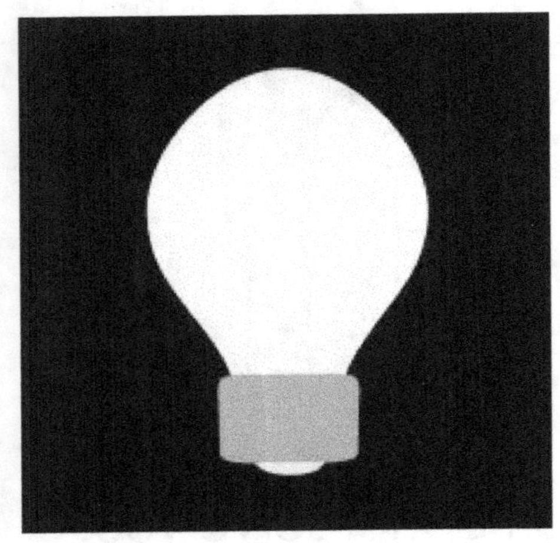

Aphasia Tips

The following list contains helpful phrases and questions patients can point to if you are able to read.

- **Please be patient.**
- **I am having trouble getting the words out.**
- **Give me a minute.**
- **I am having trouble understanding.**
- **Please use simple words.**
- **I can hear you fine. You do not need to yell.**
- **Speak slower.**
- **Please talk slower.**
- **Please repeat what you just said**
- **Call my: wife / husband/ daughter / son / mother / father / friend**
- **I understood what you said.**
- **I did not understand what you said.**
- **Please explain that again.**

- **Please do not yell. My hearing is fine.**
- **When will I see a speech therapist?**
- **How long will I be here?**
- **Why am I here?**
- **How large was my stroke? Please show me a scan of the damage.**
- **What medication are you giving me?**
- **I'd like to talk to somebody about insurance.**
- **Why did you give me thick liquids?**
- **I am thirsty.**
- **I am hungry.**
- **I need to use the bathroom.**
- **I would like to take a shower.**

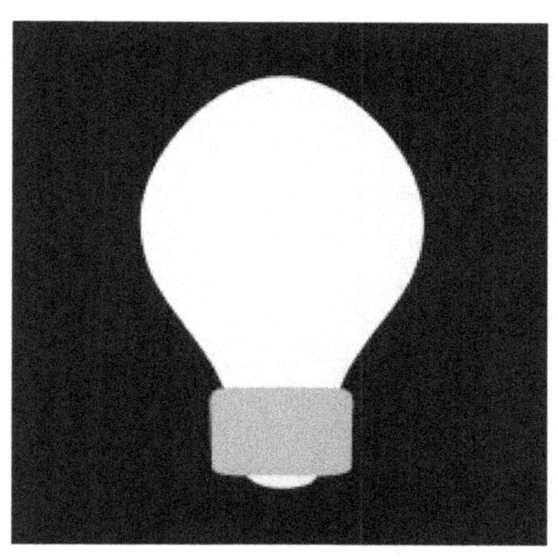

Aphasia Tip

Ask your family member to post information about you in your room. Pictures and information can help the staff know a little bit about you if you are unable to tell them.

Have somebody write down your interests and profession. Seeing a photo of you before your brain injury can go a long way helping nursing and rehab staff see you for who you are and not what your medical chart says about you.

When David was hospitalized, Carol put a poster board above his bed. She wrote:

- **David has aphasia.**
- **He is in the 4th grade.**
- **He was in the gifted program and very social.**
- **He communicates his needs by thumbs up/down for yes and no.**
- **He has difficulty understanding speech.**
- **Go slow.**
- **Keep it simple.**
- **Emphasize key words.**
- **His mom's name is Carol.**
- **His dad is Dr. James Dow**
- **His step-dad is George Richards.**
- **His brother is Michael Dow.**
- **David loves his dog, Schroder.**
- **David cannot speak, read, or write.**

Writing

Many people with aphasia are also paralyzed or have weakness in the right arm. Try using your non-dominant hand. Some people with aphasia struggle to write due to the aphasia, others don't.

At first, Carol thought David could not write because his right arm was paralyzed. Later she learned that aphasia had affected his ability to recognize letters and shapes. Today, David uses his left hand to write, tie his shoes, and even use chopsticks.

If you can, you should use it as much as possible. Writing may actually help with your recovery and will not hinder your future ability to regain verbal skills.

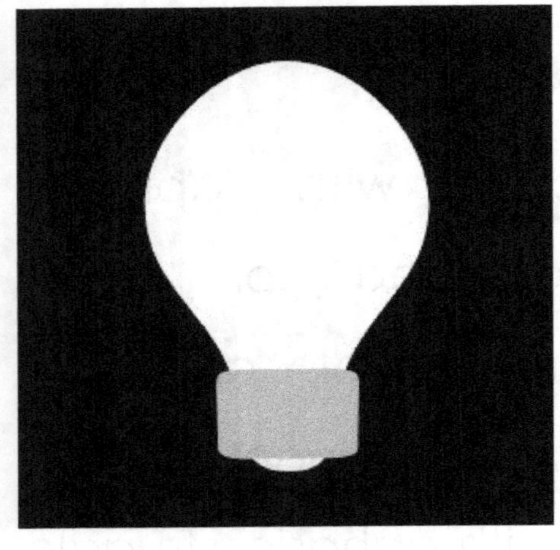

Aphasia Tip

If you haven't had a chance to see if you can write, now is the time! Call for your nurse or caregiver and point to the question below.

- ***Please bring me some paper and a pen.***

First, try writing your name. If you are able, write your name or practice writing your address, your phone number and other personal information. Are you able to write numbers? (Sometimes those are challenging in the beginning.)

Also, try writing communication phrases such as, "Hi, how are you?" Try copying the phrase: **"I have aphasia."**

Technology Tip

If you have trouble with printing with a pen and paper, most smartphones have a notepad feature. You can try typing out

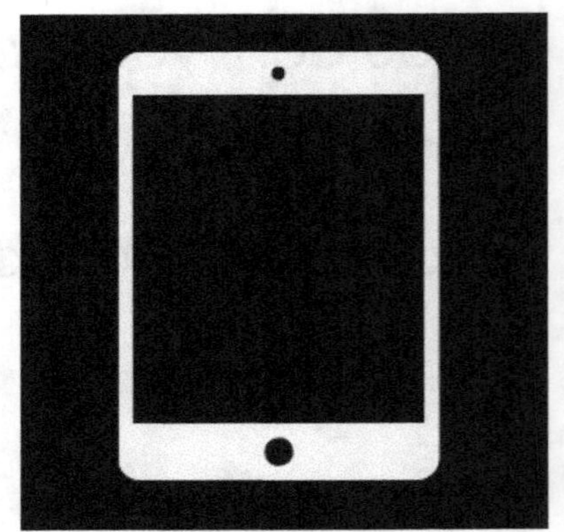

what you want to say. There are some basic apps that can even read aloud what you type. For example, Android users can try *Talk Free App* and IOS users can try *Talk For Me- Text to Speech* app. Just search "text to speech" in your app store.

What if I Have Problems Swallowing?

Difficulty swallowing is called dysphagia. As many as 65% of stroke survivors have dysphagia.[xxiii] Strokes and brain injuries can cause damage to the nerves and muscles that control

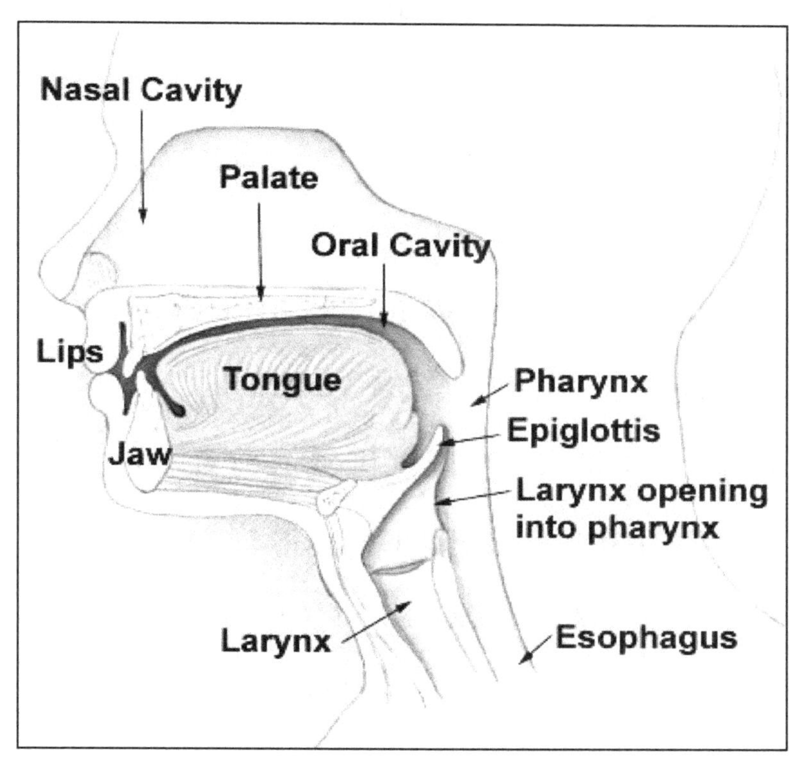

swallowing. Swallowing disorders are very serious because if you get food or liquid in your airway (trachea) and into your lungs it can cause aspiration pneumonia.

Weakened swallowing function can also result in food lodging in your airway and result in choking and possibly death.[xxiv]

Refer to this diagram to understand the swallow process. In a normal swallow, the food or bolus travels through the oral cavity until it hits the back of the tongue and triggers the swallow reflex. The epiglottis closes to protect the larynx and the bolus travels safely into the esophagus.

Stroke survivors experience a variety of dysphagia symptoms that can result in food or liquid falling into the larynx and down into the airway and lungs, which is called **aspiration**. Coughing, wet vocal quality after a swallow, tearing eyes and runny noses are all signs and symptoms of aspiration. Strokes can weaken the muscles in the throat, making it difficult to clear food out of the pharynx. Damage from a brain injury can cause the epiglottis to move slower and thin liquids (regular liquids) can spill down into the trachea before the epiglottis has completely protected the airway.

Some stroke and brain injury survivors are given the status NPO, which means "**nothing by mouth**" and need a feeding tube to safely obtain nutrition and hydration. Others will need thickened liquids in order to allow enough time to swallow safely and prevent liquids from entering your airway.

Your first encounter with a Speech-Language Pathologist (SLP) may be during a bedside swallow evaluation to determine what you can safely swallow. They may request a doctor's order for a Modified Barium Swallow (MBS), which is a video x-ray of your swallow. A MBS will show whether or not you are aspirating (food or liquids going down the wrong way).

Your SLP may offer some types of exercises to strengthen your swallowing muscles and increase your safety with swallowing. Dysphagia typically takes priority over aphasia therapy. Your SLP will focus on making sure you can eat and drink without the risk of choking or aspiration. It is a good idea to think of your SLP as a coach guiding you through the recovery process. They have the tools to teach you how to improve and they can show you what you need to do on your own to improve your swallowing.

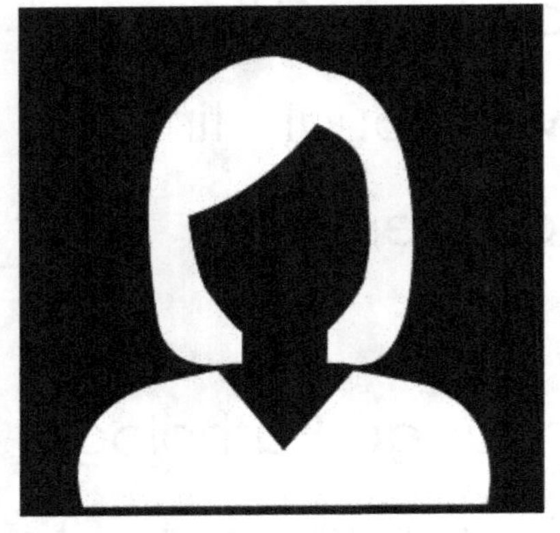

Ask your Speech Therapist (SLP):

➢ *What exercises can I do on my own to improve swallowing?*

➢ *What can I start to do on my own to improve communication?*

➢ *Can you show my family how to work with me on my goals?*

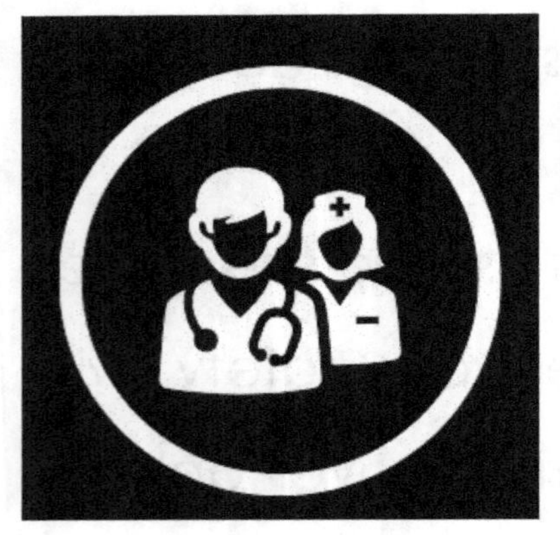

Who are All These People?
Your Recovery Team

Most hospitals have an entire rehab team dedicated to helping you recover. You may have several doctors and specialists working with you.

Neurologist: A neurologist is a stroke specialist that works to diagnose and treat the underlying stroke or other cause of aphasia. Their focus will be to reduce the damage from the stroke and help your medical team prevent any recurrent strokes.

Physical Medicine and Rehabilitation (PM&R) Doctor: This is the doctor whose role is to enhance and restore functional ability and quality of life to people with physical impairments or disabilities. They work with your rehabilitation team. Another name for this type of doctor is Physiatrist.

Physical Therapists (PTs): A PT helps with gross motor (large motor) rehabilitation. They may help with fitting with a wheelchair, walking, and keeping you safe while you adapt to any paralysis you may have.

Occupational Therapists (OTs): An OT helps with fine motor rehabilitation. They help you adapt to being one handed if you have one-sided weakness, which is called **hemiparesis**. They also work to help restore function to the use of your weakened hand and arm. OTs also work with activities of daily living such as bathing, dressing, cooking and more.

Speech-Language Pathologists (SLPs): Your Speech Therapist helps you recover your language skills of talking, reading, writing, and understanding. They can also treat swallowing disorders (dysphagia).

You and your loved ones are also big players on the team. Just like with a sports team where players work together, they are well rested when they come to "practice." When the players are motivated to do their best, the entire team benefits. Staying engaged is the way to maximize your opportunity to make the best recovery possible.

> **A very famous speech therapist, Dr. Audrey Holland, shares, "Acknowledgement is active. It permits you to be the boss of you – instead of letting aphasia be the boss of you."**

It may be helpful if family and friends do their best to reduce any stress in your life. You have enough on your plate dealing with aphasia! When someone offers your family some help, take it! A meal. A ride. Perhaps a run to the grocery store. All those tasks take time and energy – and it's best if you focus on getting better! See the caregiver chapter for more suggestions on how others can help.

What Should Visitors Know About Me and Aphasia?

Immediately after a stroke or brain injury you will be naturally tired and fatigue easily. Your body needs sleep to help repair and recover. Aphasia often worsens when you are tired or stressed.

You may be eager to see family and friends and also have some natural concerns about how they will react to your aphasia. It is helpful if they have some understanding of aphasia before their visit, especially that your language is impaired (and expected to improve) and your intellect is intact. Remember, your aphasia is likely now at its worst.

Recovery is a slow process, but you can expect to make progress with time.

Or, you may prefer to limit visitors in the beginning, which is what Carol did. She shares it was emotionally and physically draining to be living in the hospital for 3 months, but she felt that visitors would be draining. Only people who we invited were allowed. Others were told we have a "no visitor" rule and we'd love to see them when we returned home once David was stabilized and we had time to adjust to this new world of aphasia on our own first.

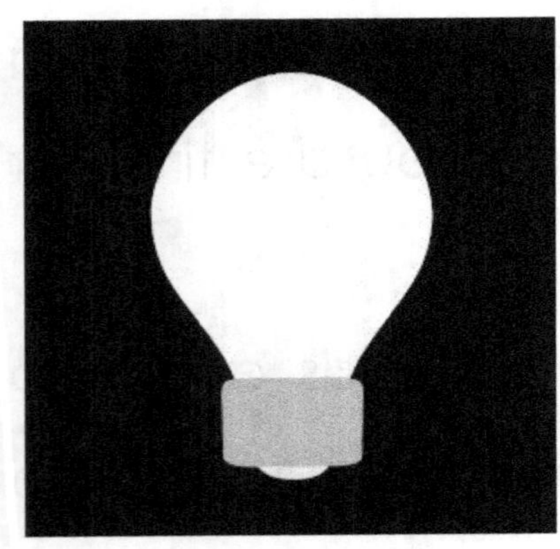

Aphasia Tips

Tips to consider when having visitors:

➤ Limit visits

➤ Be sure to include the person with aphasia in the decision-making.

➤ Reduce background noise.

➤ Keep the visits short.

➤ Turn off the TV.

- Have only one visitor at a time
- Try to avoid side conversations.
- Avoid visits before or right after therapy.
- Evenings and weekends are sometimes better for visitors.
- Ask visitors to bring photos, magazines, music or games so you can enjoy visiting with less focus on talking.
- What will help improve progress?
- What would you like to do and who would you like to see and when?

Aphasia is much more than language loss. For most people, there is a tremendous emotional struggle as they try to cope as a family with the life obstacles that come along with aphasia. Role changes, loss of job, sense of identity, financial concerns – are only a few that most families face. It is often best for the person with aphasia to have some say when they are ready to see visitors.

Having to deal with so many changes at once is unsettling. It takes time to cope and you may or may not want visitors. But do encourage visitors as soon as you feel you are ready. Practicing your speech is good for your recovery. And seeing good friends can indeed be good for the soul. You and your family will know best.

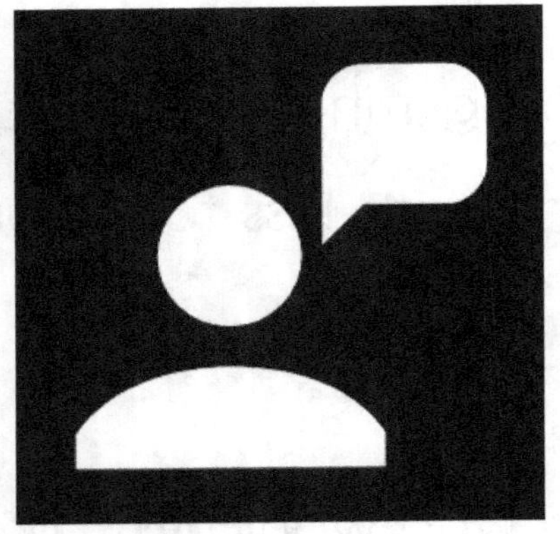

Self Evaluation:

➤ **What do I want my medical team to know about me?**

- My name is:

____

- My family members are:

____

- My friends are:

____

- What I do for work:

____

- My hobbies are:

____

- My pets are:

____

> **Who are the people on my Recovery Team?**

- Doctor: ___________________________________

- Neurologist: _______________________________

- Nurse or Nurses: ___________________________

____

- Physical Rehabilitation (PM&R) Doctor:

____

- Physical Therapist (PT): _____________________

- Occupational Therapist (OT): ________________

- Speech Therapist (SLP) ______________________

- Names of other people (family, friends, social worker):

____

____

____

Other Notes:

REHAB OPTIONS

> **What Happens When I Leave The Hospital?**

> **What Is A Rehabilitation Hospital?**

> **What Is A Skilled Nursing Facility?**

> **What Is An Assisted Living Facility?**

> **What Will Medicare Cover?**

> **What Happens When I Go Home?**

Leaving the Hospital

The severity of your stroke or injury and your physical limitations will determine where you go next and when you leave. While many patients look forward to discharge, remember, the road to recovery can be a long one. You will continue ongoing therapy and hard work to help your recovery and maintain the gains you made while in the hospital. Your discharge is just the beginning of ongoing recovery. It is important you don't stop working now!

Some people with aphasia continue speech therapy thru outpatient therapy in a facility. Others may choose telemedicine on video conferencing rather than going to a facility. Telemedicine is gaining popularity as more insurance companies now cover this type of therapy for speech.

Some patients will be discharged from an acute hospital to a rehab hospital. Others go to assisted living facilities. Some patients move to a skilled nursing home.

Often, your insurance may influence the next steps of where you go and the therapy you will receive based on your needs. Your Recovery Team will help guide you as you consider your discharge options. Sometimes a social worker may help you and your family look at options.

Knowing your insurance coverage is helpful at this time to understand the limitations of your policy. Can you travel? How many days of therapy will be covered each year? Are there limits?

The options may be limited, but you still can tell people what you need. You can ask if you can save some therapy sessions for another time if you do not use them all in the hospital. You want to ensure you maximize your benefits on a timeline that works best for your recovery within the parameters your insurer may have. Talk to your speech therapist for guidance and suggestions.

Ask your doctor and social worker to help refer you to a rehabilitation hospital if that is your next step. The social worker will help you determine what your insurance will cover.

Be honest with the hospital staff as you look at options. Do you have family dynamics or budget concerns that affect the decision? Will someone be available to take you to your rehab appointments? Are you looking to utilize insurance only benefits or are you willing to private-pay continued treatment if your insurance coverage is limited? These variables are important as well.

Let's review some of the options you may be considering once you are discharged from acute care:

In David's case, his stroke happened while on a family vacation out west. The hospital staff suggested a nearby rehab hospital that was one of the best in the country. However, the family chose to go to a rehab hospital that was closer to their home rather than be so far from family and friends.

Cost and family considerations weighed into David's family's decision. Had they opted for the "best" that would have meant 2–3 months of added hotel, transportation, and food costs as well as being away from home. David had a brother at home that Carol needed to care for too, and she had a business. It was not practical, and they had to face that reality.

What is a Rehabilitation Hospital?

Rehab hospitals are devoted to patients who have stabilized their medical issues and are approved for continued care and services within an inpatient medical setting. Often they are separate facilities, but occasionally they are units within a larger hospital.

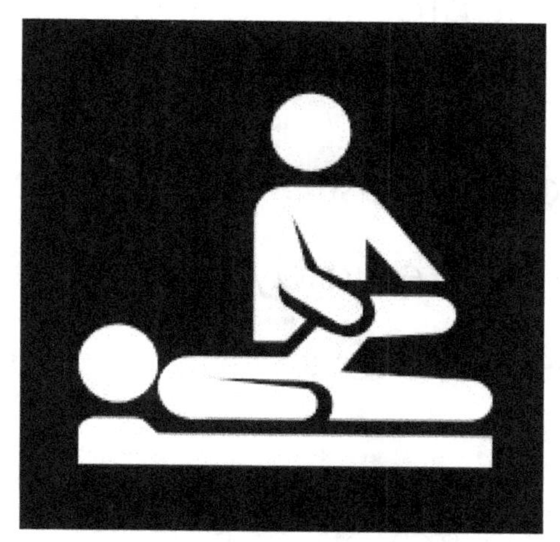

While you may choose the recommendation the staff makes, also remember that you have a choice where you go for rehabilitation. Of course, your insurance carrier also may impact that decision.

You and your family are your own advocates.

There are rehabilitation hospitals with special units devoted solely to stroke and brain injury rehabilitation. Even if you need to travel, it maybe worth the inconvenience of a day or more of travel to reach the best rehabilitation team for your needs.

U.S News and World Report ranks the best rehabilitation hospitals in the country. In 2019-2020 their top six were:

1. Shirley Ryan AbilityLab, Chicago (Formally Rehabilitation Institute of Chicago)

2. Spaulding Rehabilitation Hospital, Charlestown, MA

3. TIRR Memorial Hermann in Houston, TX4. Kessler Institute for Rehabilitation in West Orange, NJ

5. University of Washington Medical Center in Seattle, WA

6. Mayo Clinic in Rochester, MN[xxv]

The *U.S. News and World Report* website has more rankings of rehabilitation hospitals. There may be one located much closer to you on the list. US News and World Report list.

www.sci-info-pages.com/top-rehabilitation-hospitals/

What is a Skilled Nursing Facility?

A skilled nursing facility (SNF) cares for patients who need long-term nursing care or rehabilitation therapy services. Sometimes it is called a long-term care facility, nursing home, or rehab center.

If you have multiple medical needs and require physical, occupational, and speech therapy, a skilled nursing facility may be a good option. You may have a choice in where you go for therapy. If you can, have a friend or loved one visit several to help you decide.

Most patients with strokes and aphasia do continue to improve and you'll want to maintain the motivation to keep working hard in therapy to eventually be discharged to a lower level of care facility or even home!

Questions to Ask a Skilled Nursing Facility

If you have someone tour skilled nursing facilities for you, there are some important things they should look for and questions they might ask on your behalf.

➢ How many hours a week can you expect to get therapy?

➢ How many years of experience does the Speech-Language Pathologist have? Are they a Certified First Year (CFY)? **CFY** means the speech therapist is in their first year out of graduate school. Sometimes this can be a positive thing because new graduates are typically full of energy and will be motivated to give you the best therapy they can. On the flip side, CFYs may lack the experience that may be necessary for your ideal rehabilitation.

➢ Do they use graduate student clinicians? This will mean a student could be the one treating you, then reporting to a supervisor.

➢ Does the speech therapist give homework assignments?

➢ Can family members or close friends participate in therapy?

➢ Are there other patients at the SNF with aphasia who would be interested in doing carryover speech therapy communication activities together?

➢ What type of guidance do they give their patients once they leave the skilled nursing setting?

➢ Do they provide a care plan for you once you return home? Some skilled nursing facilities will have the physical and/or occupational therapist visit your home and do a safety evaluation before you move back home. This is a good sign that they help you with the transition back home.

➤ What training has the staff had in the last 12 months on aphasia? Communication access is a human right and the quality of your care is dependent on others having an understanding of aphasia and their ability to interact with you.

When visiting a skilled nursing facility (SNF), try to meet with the social or activities director. Some SNFs have an excellent working relationship between the therapy and activities department. Goals for aphasia can be carried over into activities throughout the day with the activity and nursing staff. Staying active and engaged is key for your recovery – and your well-being.

More Questions to Ask a Skilled Nursing Facility

There are also other things to look for when you have somebody visit a skilled nursing facility:

- When touring a room, pull the safety call bell. See how long it takes the nursing staff to get to that room to make sure the resident is safe.
- Try to view a meal, does it look appealing?
- Are the residents engaged with others?
- How much supervision and help do the residents receive?
- Is the facility clean? Does the nursing staff seem content and happy?
- Are the residents involved in activities and up and about?
- Is the environment helpful to your aphasia?
- Is it quiet or full of noise and distractions?
- Do they have other patients with aphasia?
- What communication supports are they using?

Hopefully, you will have a chance to tour multiple facilities and pick the one that is the best fit for both nursing and rehabilitation. Sometimes, time and distance from home may be a deciding factor.

Unlike a rehabilitation hospital not everybody who resides at a skilled nursing center is destined to return home. Many patients live there on a long-term basis and have progressive conditions that will only get worse such as advanced dementia or Alzheimer's. It is important that the staff understand your type of aphasia. You might want to post information up on the wall, like we suggested earlier.

Sadly, other patients' conditions may be important to you when deciding where to go for rehabilitation. It could impact your emotional health to be in a skilled nursing facility because of the nature of some of the other patients' conditions. Try to find one that supports your aphasia with a bright, cheery atmosphere that supports your own well-being.

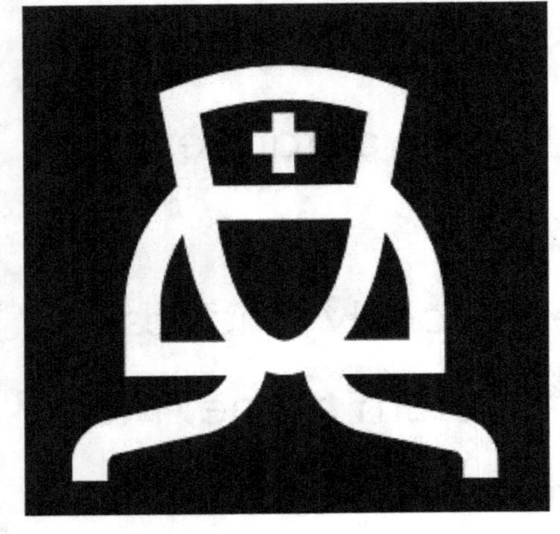

Assisted Living Facilities

Assisted Living Facilities (ALFs) are residential buildings for people who require a variety of assistance throughout the day. ALFs provide meals, medical care, and assistance with activities of daily living. Some may have their own rehabilitation departments, eliminating the need to travel to outpatient therapy. Sometimes assisted living facilities are a transition between skilled nursing and home. If you have limited medical needs, an assisted living facility may be a good fit for you.

Assisted living would be a good fit for somebody who was thinking about moving to a place with additional support before their stroke or brain injury. If moving back home and living alone causes you and your family concern, assisted living could be the solution.

Carol's dad, also a stroke survivor, resides in an ALF and is socially engaged and has made many friends. It was a big adjustment at first, but he'd be the first to tell you it was a very good decision and he's happy with the social life it has offered him.

If you are considering assisted living, have someone meet with the rehab director for you if you can't do it yourself.

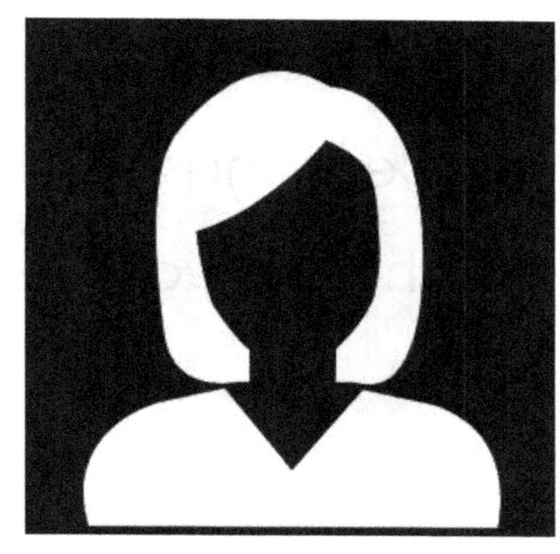

Questions to ask Speech Therapist at the ALF

Some ALFs have speech therapists. When visiting an assisted living facility, meet with the speech therapist. *You can ask these questions:*

> *How many treatments will you have?*

> *How long are the treatment times?*

> *Are there any volunteers that come to the facility?*

> *Are they available to help with communication goals between therapy sessions?*

Review the activity schedule and try to get a feel for how active and social the other residents are. Do they have activities you would like to participate in? You may not feel like it at first, as you have a lot to cope with. But, with time you may find yourself connecting with others in a safe environment and find yourself quite content.

When touring the facility, make a note if the marketing director shows off the rehabilitation department or if they only mention it briefly. Ideally, you want a place that is proud of their therapy department and understands that their residents benefit greatly from all of the services it provides.

Some of the best information you will receive is from current patients.

> Do they look content?

> Do they like the food?

> If you can visit over mealtime, do the patients seem engaged and cared for?

Sometimes, talking to residents will give you a better sense of care than the marketing representative. It is their job to fill rooms – but it is your job to ensure a good fit. Don't be shy to ask questions, as this is a very important decision.

Home Health

If you are able to go home, you may have the option of having therapists coming to you. If it is difficult for you to travel to and from appointments, you may qualify for home health therapy. Home health can work with you on communication challenges that you experience.

Home care is care that is provided in your own home by licensed medical professionals such as a speech, physical, or music therapists. It may also include assistance provided by a professional caregiver for needs such as bathing or activities of daily living.

Most home health speech therapists are paid by the visit and not by the time spent with you. They receive the same reimbursement whether they spend 15 minutes or an hour with you. Home health therapists often have to complete lengthy forms for every visit.

Having speech therapy sessions in your home can help with real life situations and communicating with family and friends. It is also helpful to have therapy at home if you find fatigue is an issue. If you have obstacles getting to an outpatient clinic, home health can be a wonderful option.

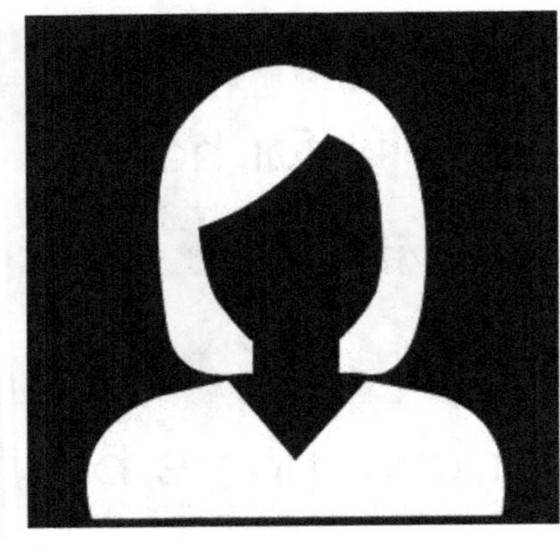

Before you select a therapist ask the therapist these questions:

> ➤ ***What are the time commitments and expectations?***

> ➤ ***Can my family and / or friends help with my therapy?***

> ➤ ***Will you give me homework to work on outside of therapy?***

> ➤ ***Can I share my goals? And make it custom for my interests?***

Outpatient Therapy

Outpatient therapy is an option for people who are able to live at home but still need ongoing rehabilitation. Outpatient therapy clinics are available in a variety of

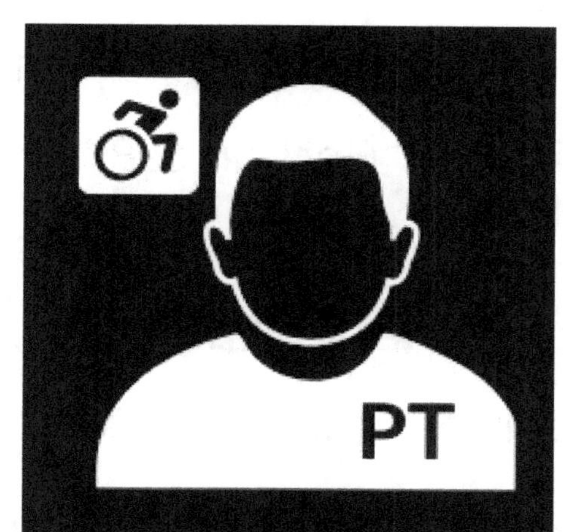

settings but often you will find that your options are limited by your insurance coverage.

Hospitals often have a separate outpatient rehabilitation clinic. Skilled nursing facilities have rehabilitation departments and sometimes are happy to see patients on an outpatient basis. Private practice speech therapy offices are also an option. Some private practices appear to only treat pediatric patients, but it could be worth your time to call and see if they also see adult patients or if they specialize in aphasia therapy.

Since your insurance may limit the number of visits you have with your speech therapist, finding an appropriate therapist for your aphasia is important. Key factors in selecting your speech therapist would include ensuring that they treat adults and have experience with aphasia therapy. To find a speech therapist (also known as an SLP, Speech-Language Pathologist) that is certified by the American Speech-Language-Hearing Association, visit https://www.asha.org/findpro/ and click on "Find an SLP."

David went to speech therapy from age 10 to age 25. During that time, he had many different speech therapists. Some he liked. Some he didn't. He liked the ones who challenged him and believed in him. Just like any profession, you will find some you like, some you don't. Some are good with a lot of experience in aphasia. Others have little to no experience with aphasia.

What Are Telepractice and Other Virtual Options?

Telepractice refers to any type of therapy linking the clinician and patient through telecommunications

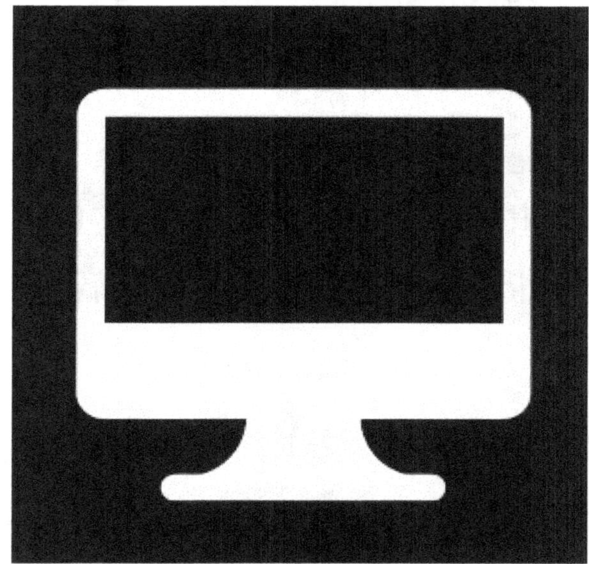

technology. [xxvi] The American Speech-Language-Hearing Association (ASHA) has approved telepractice as an acceptable form of treatment. Many people with aphasia enjoy teletherapy as they don't have to go to a clinic to receive speech therapy services and the caregiver is often relieved of driving to and from appointments.

Additionally, patients can find speech therapists that specialize in aphasia therapy rather than the nearest therapist who may or may not have had much experience with aphasia. Remember, it is your recovery.

You matter. Ask questions. You and your insurance are the payers and it is perfectly fine for you to speak up and ensure you are getting what you need.

Amanda (this book's co-author) sees her aphasia patients via teletherapy. Some therapists are licensed in multiple states. To learn more, check out Amanda's website at: aphasiateletherapy.com.

There are multiple aphasia treatment centers that offer aphasia treatment via telepractice. Not all insurance companies pay for telepractice so you should verify to make sure it is covered. Since the COVID-19 Pandemic some insurance carriers have approved reimbursement for teletherapy that previously was not covered.

Some people opt to cash pay for additional therapy if insurance has stopped covering. Do not believe (even for an instant!) that just because insurance stopped – you should stop your efforts!

Virtual options for aphasia are expanding. Support groups, including ARC, have expanded their remote group options post COVID-19. ARC offers daily opportunities for people with aphasia and caregivers to connect with their program Virtual Connections.

These sessions are facilitated by aphasia therapists, music therapists, and other experts on video conferencing. Often, you'll meet 10-20 other people with aphasia on a call. There are offered FREE. Learn how by going here: https://devices.aphasia.com/virtual-connections

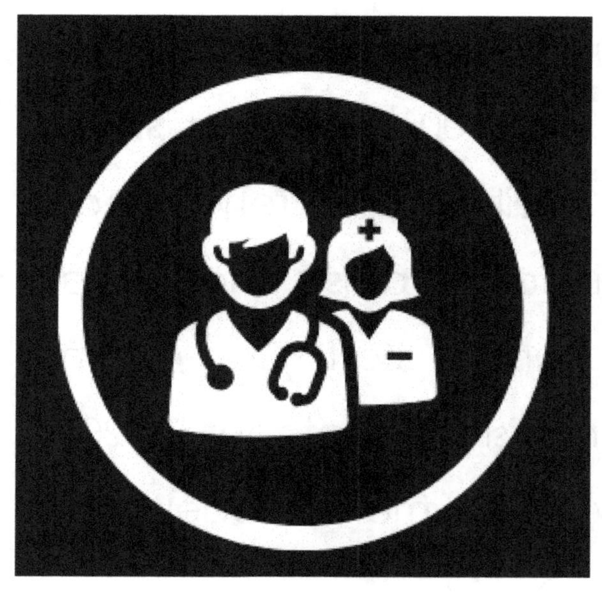

Clinical Trials

Another way to get the most out of your therapy is to participate in clinical research trials. This is a way to obtain free therapy to improve your communication abilities. Visit: https://clinicaltrials.gov Type the word "aphasia" in the search box. You can search trials by location to see if there are any studies near you.

Questions for Insurance and Medicare
What Does Medicare or Insurance Cover?

Note: This applies to the US options available at the time of publication, but if you live in other places check your local options.

At the time of publication (2020), if you have Medicare, Part A covers the cost of your first 100 days in a **skilled nursing facility**. A skilled nursing facility has a rehab team with physical therapists, occupational therapists and speech therapists in addition to a full nursing staff. One of the benefits of staying in a SNF is that since October 1, 2019 Medicare instituted patient driven payment model there are no longer time limitations on therapy.

If you have Medicare and choose **assisted living** you will most likely use your Medicare part B benefits to cover therapy. Medicare Part B covers 80% of therapy costs at this time.

In 2018, the U.S. Congress passed a new law that removed therapy caps for Medicare Part B patients. The therapy caps were replaced with a targeted medical review threshold of $3,000 for speech and physical therapy combined and $3,000 for occupational therapy. [xxvii] This means that once your therapy has reached $3,000 in costs for both physical and speech therapy your therapists will need to document additional medical necessity information on their Medicare Part B claims. This is an improvement from past set Medicare Part B caps, which sometimes prevented patients from getting the therapy they needed. Medicare.gov states "Medicare law no longer limits how much it pays for your medically necessary outpatient therapy services in one calendar year."[xxviii]

Therapy benefits are allotted for each calendar year. Often your insurance benefits for speech therapy may run out after the first three months. Keep this in mind when you are working with your Speech-Language Pathologist. You can remind them that you need goals and activities to help you through the remainder of the year if you need to space out your therapy sessions over time because you are concerned about coverage limitations. Or, ask if they are planning to advocate on your behalf to get more therapy.

Sometimes you do have to be the advocate and push just a little, and that is OK. Your recovery matters! Be kind and helpful. Ask if there is anything you (or your loved one) can do to assist.

Carol became a fierce advocate for David's therapy. One of her tactics was to call the insurance and find out how the insurance company would be willing to expand therapy. (You may find it online these days.) Then, she wrote down word for word the exact language the insurance company used. She gave the information to the doctor and therapists and asked them to use those parameters when they contacted the insurance company.

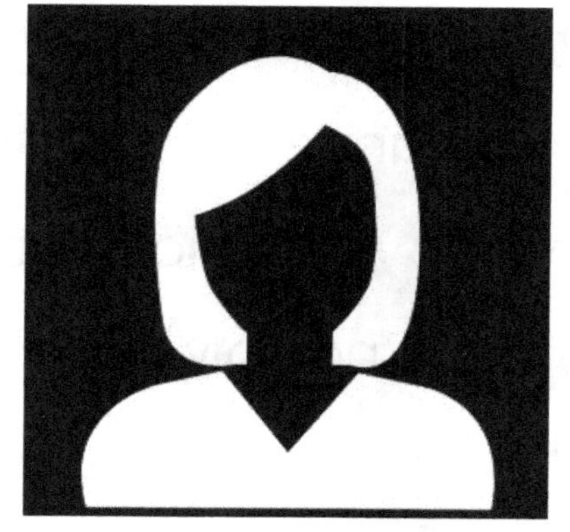

Questions you can ask your SLP:

➤ *What can I do on my own once my therapy benefits run out?*

➤ *Could you make me a treatment plan for the rest of the year?*

➤ *Are there therapy apps specific to my type of aphasia you would recommend?*

When a new calendar year begins, your therapy benefits reset. This is the time to begin therapy again, which will require a new physician's prescription. Sometimes, patients are treated once a week in order to ration therapy for the entire year. This may be considered a "red flag" for insurance denial because it may appear to be maintenance therapy, which is usually not covered. Once you begin therapy at the beginning of each year, try to leave with a plan to keep yourself going throughout the year. The best way to ensure more coverage is to work hard and show gains. Just going to therapy and not engaging is more likely to result in no gains – and insurance will not continue.

Sometimes family members find that advocating and being the "squeaky wheel" with the insurance company, doctor, and therapist may result in an extension and approval for more services. However, this is not always the case because sometimes there are strict insurance limits on access to ongoing therapy.

Remember to check all options with your insurance so you do not have any surprises.

Some Final Thoughts
on Facilities and Therapy Options

No matter what therapy and facility you choose or even if you can go home -- we have found that motivation is key to a successful recovery. We believe it is important that there is a good connection between you and your Speech-Language Pathologist. If you find yourself in a situation where you struggle to connect, it is your responsibility to self-advocate and seek out another therapist. In fact, sometimes switching is a good idea—as every therapist brings fresh ideas and approaches.

These steps from discharge to home, a facility, or other options can feel overwhelming. But these decisions are key o your ongoing optimal recovery. Get a notebook andstart to weigh out your options, check your insurance, and perhaps check with the social worker if you are still in the hospital at the time you are reading this guide.

David offers this advice, "If your therapist doesn't believe in you and your ability to progress and you are motivated, you can ask to change therapists. I did best with the ones that specialized in aphasia and who knew how to keep challenging me at the right level. But the most important person in therapy is you and your own motivation, determination, and persistence."

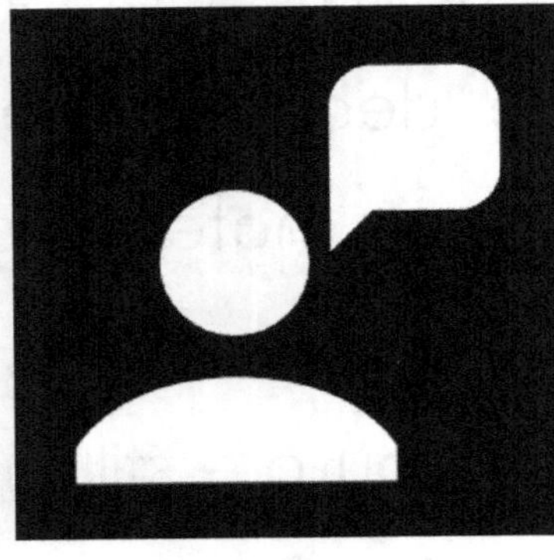

Self Evaluation:

➤ **What should I (or my family member)**

➤ **ask about my choices when I leave the hospital?**

____

____

➤ **Notes on Therapy Options:**

____

____

____

____

____

➤ **Notes on Insurance Coverage:**

____

____

____

____

➢ **What would work best for my family? Do you live alone? Do you live with someone**

____

____

____

____

Other Notes:

- ➢ **How Can My Family Help With My Recovery?**
- ➢ **What Can My Friends Do To Help?**
- ➢ **How Can I Connect With Other People?**
- ➢ **How Do I Build A Support Team?**
- ➢ **What Groups Are Helpful?**
- ➢ **How Can I Stay Active?**

What is My Family Thinking?

Friends and family of someone with aphasia often want to help, but sometimes are at a loss when it comes to knowing what to do or even having a good understanding of aphasia, as it is indeed a very complex and misunderstood disorder. Sadly, although aphasia affects over two million in the US, most people have no idea what aphasia is. That further increases the challenges you may face.

Since aphasia is a communication disorder, it is a challenge for people with aphasia to communicate their needs and best strategies. Concerned family and friends sometimes mistake the inability to talk for indifference, the desire of the person with aphasia to be left alone, or mistaken for just being difficult and "not trying." Or worse, others may believe that aphasia has affected your intellect or perhaps you are impaired by drugs or alcohol.

A person with aphasia still can form their own thoughts and opinions; they just have trouble communicating what they are. You are still smart.

Staying active will help your recovery. Engaging with friends and activities is very good for you. But, it will be important that those around you understand your condition and learn ways to be supportive.

How Can My Family Help with My Recovery?

It is helpful for families to learn the skills needed to become an effective communication partner. Aphasia happened not only to you, but to those you love as well. Communication affects so many aspects of your life and there is a lot of coping that needs to happen. It is not uncommon for there to be rough days for both you and your family. *Everyone* needs to adjust to the challenges aphasia brings.

Your first level of support will likely come from family. In some cases a family member will become your Power of Attorney. Not because you are intellectually incapable of managing your medical care, but because you may need somebody to help communicate your wants and needs. A Power of Attorney is someone who legally acts on your behalf in financial, medical, or legal matters.

Be careful not to let your pride prevent family members from helping you.

Speech-Language Pathologists encounter all types of family dynamics. Some people with aphasia struggle with letting family manage some of their medical and financial affairs. It is important that your family member acknowledges that your intelligence is intact and that they review important decisions with you.

On the opposite end, be aware of the condition of **learned helplessness**. Sometimes it is easy to give up and let somebody else do everything for you just because they are willing. Make sure you continue doing things you are capable of even if it is a challenge and takes longer than usual. Letting someone else do things for you that you are capable of doing yourself will make the path to recovery much harder.

Aphasia recovery is not like breaking a bone and waiting for it to heal. We all wish there was a magic pill. Or a surgery to repair aphasia. There is not. Instead, you will find that recovery will take a lot of work on your part. And also from those who love you. There will be days you will not want to work hard. That is normal. Some people regain much of the their prior skills. Others are left with chronic aphasia. We want you to aim to be the best YOU can be. Start with small goals and realize it takes a very long time to see the gains for your efforts.

One of the sayings Carol keeps on her desk is this: "Successful people do what needs to be done, whether they feel like it or not." The same is true for recovery. Being successful requires getting the job done even if you don't really feel like it. The choice is yours.

> "Recovery is like a very long, long run; a marathon. It is not quick, like a sprint. You need to be patient with yourself. Others need to be patient. And you need to keep going. A runner who stops when they no longer feel motivated does not get to the finish line. Sometimes they rest. But they pick up and keep going. Work every day. Keep going." – David Dow

Often, the family is highly motivated and everyone wants you to push hard to recover. At the same time everyone needs to be reminded that what you are going through is extremely difficult. Motivation will naturally be difficult at times, especially in the beginning when you are struggle to face the new reality you find yourself in. It is common for sadness and perhaps depression to set in and interfere with your motivation. On top of that, it is very hard for you to express your feelings.

When family members offer empathy and encouragement, it is helpful. But even family members will have their limits some days. It is hard on the entire family unit. Be patient. And try not to overwhelm each other. Show appreciation and love to your caregiver too. While you are the one with aphasia, it has greatly impacted your loved one too.

What Can My Friends Do to Help?

Good friends are often eager to help you, but need to know what they can do to help. It might be uncomfortable for them at first to interact with you because you can't communicate the same way you could in the past. Some friends may be great to help you with therapy goals. You may enjoy friendships and do things together that are not as challenging to your communication needs.

Sadly, sometimes people lose friends once they have aphasia. ARC members share that their friends don't "get it." It is hard to understand aphasia and public awareness is dismal at best. Sometimes educating your friends (or perhaps your loved one can help) may bridge the gap a bit. Having strong supportive friendship patterns prior to aphasia can be helpful."[xxix]

It is unfortunate that people with aphasia are sometimes considered confused, mentally impaired, using drugs or alcohol, or having dementia. Not being able to answer orientation questions about the date and your location because of aphasia is much different than being confused and having dementia. Sometimes friends do not understand. Educating others with factual information is key so that others do not make incorrect assumptions.

Appendix E has some helpful tips for friends and family to help educate them.

Aphasia Tips

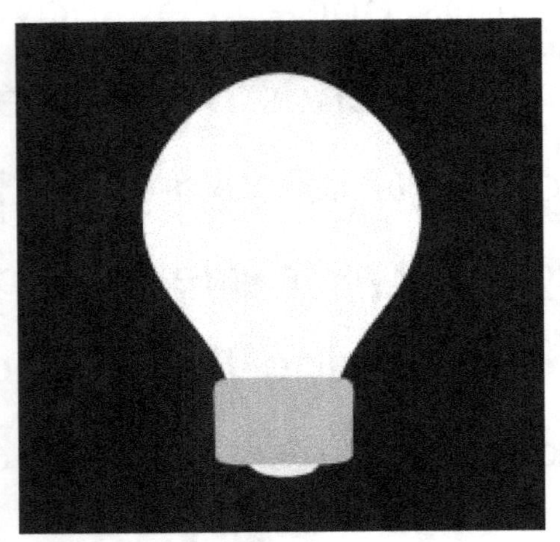

When your friends come to visit you, let them know you are still the same person inside.

> **I am the same inside but I am having trouble communicating.**

> **Slow down so I can process what you are saying.**

> **I am thinking but I have trouble speaking.**

> **Some activities that you might try later in your recovery may include:**

- o listening to music together
- o listening to an audio book
- o playing cards
- o playing board games.

What are some games that don't require much speaking?

- checkers
- chess
- bridge
- poker
- Rummikube®
- Connect Four
- Monopoly.

Pick something that you enjoyed playing before your stroke or brain injury.

What are games for building communication skills?

o Taboo

o Catch Phrase

o Heads up

o Charades

o Pictionary

o Scrabble®

o Anomia

o Scattergories

o Guess Who

While these games may be a challenge at first, all are excellent choices as language-building games. Some of them may be quite difficult, but if you have a friend you feel comfortable with and is patient with you, it is definitely a great idea to try some of these games together. Ask your speech therapist if you are ready for any of these suggestions. We want you to find success and build on that, so you want to try when you are ready to re-build the skills needed for playing games.

ARC has partnered with Carnegie Mellon, University of Pittsburgh, and Thorny Games to design games for people with aphasia. They are developing games specific to aphasia. They have brought together speech therapists, game designers, and people with aphasia. Together, they are studying game design and testing games for aphasia. Check it out! Learn more at:

www.aphasiagamesforhealth.com

Aphasia can be isolating and lonely because of the inability to communicate. Friendships are important so do your best to stay connected.

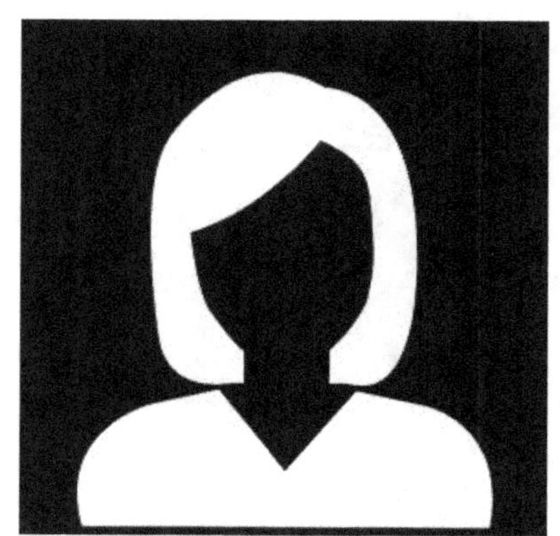

Ask your SLP for suggestions based on your current abilities.

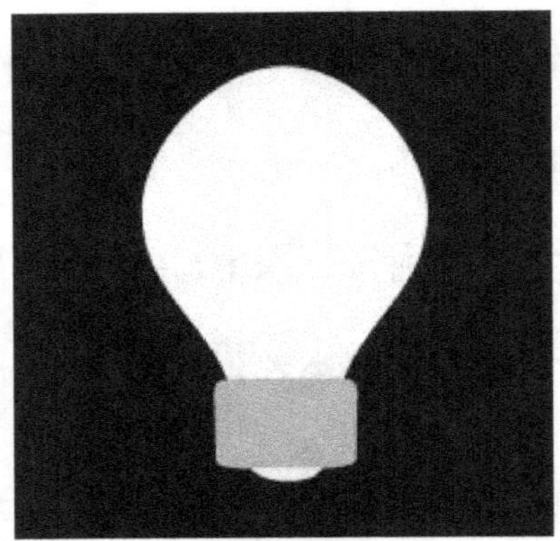

Aphasia Tips

If your friend visits and is not sure what you can do together, here are some things you can suggest:

> ➤ *Show me pictures on your smartphone.*
>
> ➤ *Please bring an easy game for us to play.*
>
> ➤ *Let's watch a favorite movie.*
>
> ➤ *Please bring your pet for a visit.*
>
> ➤ *Let's go out for coffee.*
>
> ➤ *Let's go out to lunch.*
>
> ➤ *I'd like to go to a park and get some fresh air.*
>
> ➤ *Let's go shopping together.*

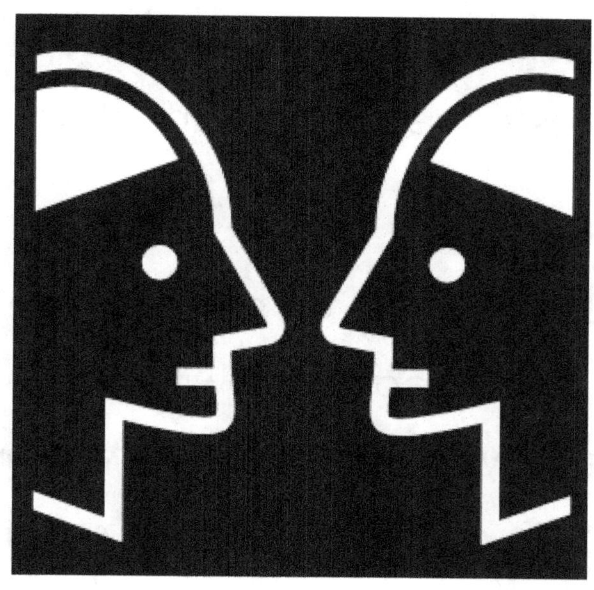

Connecting

Connecting with others is important to our well-being as humans. Having a stroke and aphasia can feel overwhelming and like a rollercoaster, but keeping your connection with old friends as well as building new relationships with those who share the same challenges and experiences can often be helpful to maintain hope and optimism.

As a nonprofit organization, Aphasia Recovery Connection works to help connect people by offering opportunities for people to meet online or offline. Much of their work is done right on Facebook, so they are easy to find. Facebook allows a place to meet others, watch videos, chat in Messenger Rooms, and so much more.

One husband of a person with aphasia shared, "I never heard my wife laugh after her stroke. One day I heard her laughing in another room. I went to check on her and saw her talking to an ARC member on a video call. The two women were struggling to get their words out but there was a connection between them. It was so heartwarming to see my wife smiling once again. Even laughing."

David, and over two million other people in the United States know the isolation aphasia brings. ARC works to bring people together, to find hope, share experiences, and help end the isolation for those who are recovering from aphasia. ARC includes learning, sharing, and most importantly – connecting you with other families dealing with aphasia. (See Chapter 11.)

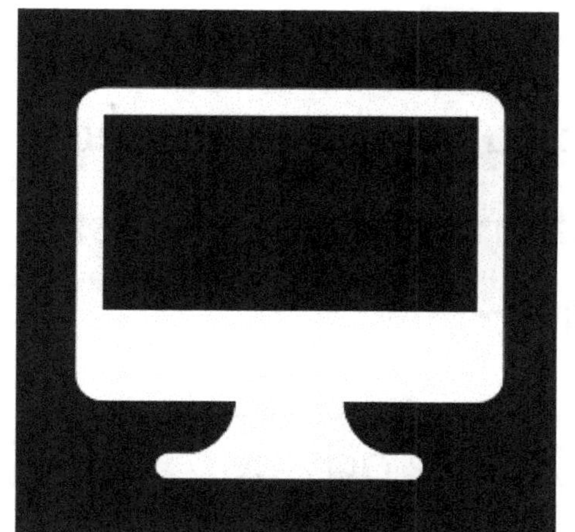

Virtual Connections

Virtual Connections is a free online meetup for families living with aphasia. Sessions are facilitated by speech-language pathologists, music therapists, and aphasia experts. People with aphasia join the sessions to meet others, share ideas, and practice communication skills. There are also sessions for care partners each week. The program offers a huge variety each week to select from. Learn more and register for a session at:

Aphasiarecoveryconnection.org/virtualconnections

How Do I Build a Support Team?

Carol was fortunate to have a strong support network when David had his stroke. Her good friend was a family therapist who had gone through a similar situation years earlier when her husband sustained a brain injury.

Most people with aphasia are in for a long road ahead and many life changes. It is a difficult time and it is best if you enlist the help of those who are willing.

Carol's friend shared this valuable advice, "When people call and ask if there is anything they can do, your answer should be, "Yes!'" As a caregiver, she appreciated those who offered to help, whether it be picking up groceries or running an errand. While is may be hard to ask for help, most of those that offer truly do want to support you on this journey, so learn to say, "Yes."

You may be surprised by the amount of people in your life and in your community who are eager to help you. Do not be afraid or too proud to ask! You can use social media to reach out to your friends and family and ask for help. Your family members can reach out to your church, school, friends, family, and even local community centers to ask for volunteers to help you with your therapy goals.

In the Caregiver Chapter 10 we cover some ideas that friends and extended family can help with outside of your aphasia therapy needs.

Remember, friends do want to help. They just aren't sure how. While it is easy to be disappointed when they don't reach out, it is also for you or your loved one to reach out to them. It doesn't hurt to ask them to help your recovery your language skills with social engagement.

Speech therapy sessions may only be 1-2 hours of your week. If you want to optimize recovery and are motivated, we suggest you find challenging and therapeutic activities to supplement your clinical therapy hours. You will learn more in the next chapter about some great options when we discuss technology.

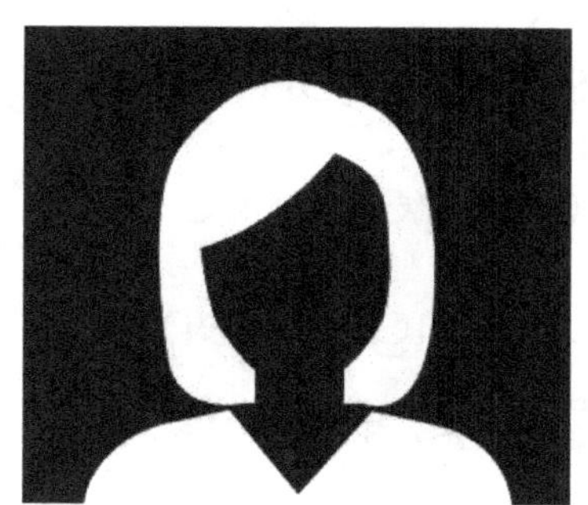

Ask your SLP

➢ *Can you provide exercises and goals that family and friends can help me with?*

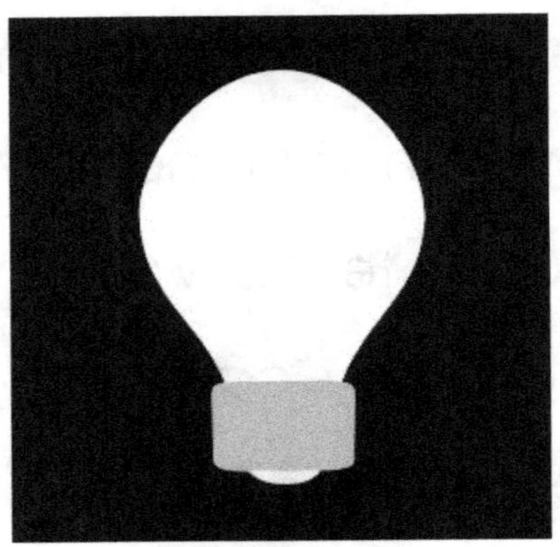

Aphasia Tips

Your family can help coordinate volunteers to come help you with communication goals.

Speech therapist Maura Silverman founded Triangle Aphasia Project in Raleigh, NC, an organization that helps people with aphasia utilize their community to increase their rehabilitation potential. They provide guidelines for therapy and have volunteers to help people get the most out of their recovery. They encourage people with aphasia to form a circle of support and reach out to their community to ask for help.

Maura encourages people with aphasia to remember that many people want to help with the recovery process, but are unsure of how to help. Engaging them in communication tasks will increase their understanding of aphasia, while helping the person with aphasia gain confidence to return to social, vocational, and recreational pursuits. A guided program allows for accessible language support and puts the ownership of the recovery process where it belongs, in the hands of the person with aphasia.

The program supports people where they live, within their own interests, and help them build a support system for success!

There are many Aphasia Centers throughout the USA that we have listed in the Appendix C. If you live near a center, we encourage you to visit and meet others with aphasia. There, you will meet leaders like Maura. You'll be glad you did! So many of these programs are led by committed and passionate aphasia leaders. They do not feel like the hospital. In fact, many centers begin to feel more like a "family" too. Do check them out!

Aphasia Recovery Connection offers many videos and opportunities online for others to learn more about aphasia. Many friends and families of those with aphasia also share their experiences and challenges on Facebook, which is a way to learn from others who are walking in your shoes. There is no 'right' or 'wrong' way to approach things; what is important is to base the choices on the person with aphasia and your own family dynamics.

What Groups Are Helpful?

There are two kinds of support groups you may wish to try. Support groups are safe places to meet others with aphasia and share your stories both online and in your community.

Aphasia Support Groups are a great way to increase the amount of time you socialize and challenge yourself. These

meetings can provide emotional reinforcement by simply letting you share and hear others' stories. In these safe settings remember to challenge yourself and talk - even if you know you may make mistakes.

Stroke Support Groups often offer these benefits as well. There may be less emphasis on aphasia. Sometimes, the facilitator may not have had communication support training, so it's a good time for you or your loved one to teach others about aphasia and topics often focus on nutrition, paralysis, coping, and community services.

Aphasia Recovery Connection is an award winning nonprofit that offers connections through Facebook for meeting others as you work on recovery. Even if you have never joined Facebook before, we suggest joining for aphasia specific support and connection. ARC's Facebook group offers you a connection to people with aphasia who are facing similar challenges and experiences.

Knowing you are not alone in your struggle can be powerful and healing. At the time of publication there were over 10,000 ARC members. ARC also posts questions and videos to help members with aphasia practice reading, writing, and comprehension. You can find ARC at this web address:

www.facebook.com/groups/Aphasia.Recovery.Connect ion/

The National Stroke Association awarded the Aphasia Recovery Connection a RAISE Award for making an impact on stroke survivors. Connection is powerful, especially for people who may have lost jobs or friends as they deal with this devastating and often misunderstood disability.

The National Aphasia Association (NAA) is another good resource for support. They provide a variety of information about aphasia for both people with the condition as well as their caregivers. By clicking Aphasia.org it will help you search for local support groups around the United States. These local support groups provide an opportunity to increase communication skills and  share with others. They are often led by a Speech-Language Pathologist.

The American Speech-Language-Hearing (ASHA) is yet another valuable resource for individuals with aphasia. You can visit them at (asha.org) to find a local graduate or undergraduate speech-language therapy program near you. Look for "Find an Education Program" on their site. Most graduate programs offer clinics to the public at a very low cost. Even if you are currently in therapy, take advantage of the extra therapy and sign up. Often it is hard for graduate programs to find enough adults for their students' clinical hours. They will be happy to have the opportunity to work with you. In fact, that is how David Dow and author Amanda met over ten years ago, patient and student clinician.

If there isn't a graduate program near your home, recruit local high school students who are looking for volunteer hours.

Four years after David's stroke, Carol found a student volunteer from a local Catholic school that required volunteer hours. The student was grateful for the opportunity to work with David and added the experience to his college application. They worked together with aphasia workbooks, reading, and played games that were all very therapeutic for David.

David's therapist assisted with the selection of materials, which ensured they were working at levels that were adequate for David. Later, Carol purchased a computer and the two began working together playing games or doing artistic projects on the computer, which David enjoyed.

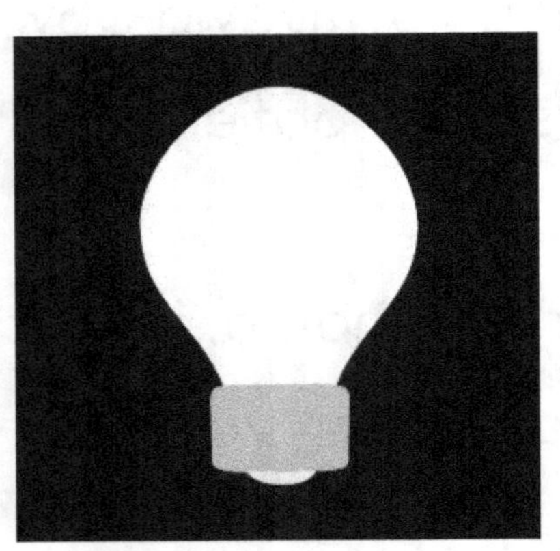

Aphasia Tips

- ➤ Look for opportunities to volunteer
- ➤ Join new groups
- ➤ Stay active in past hobbies or start new ones
- ➤ Set Goals

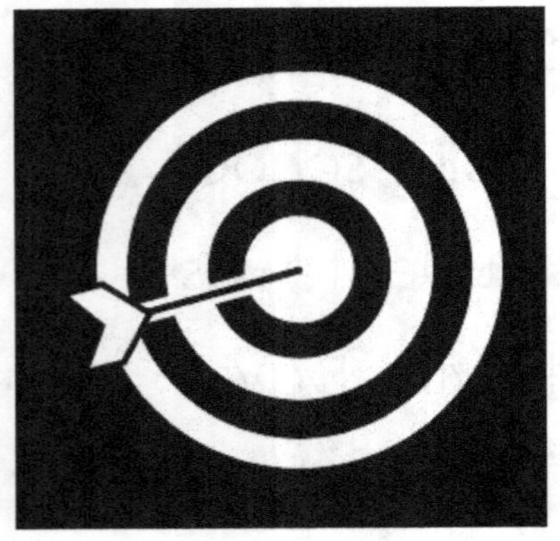

Setting Goals

Everybody needs goals and something to keep busy and the therapeutic benefits are huge. The worst thing you can do is isolate yourself, cut off interaction with the world and stay on the couch watching TV. There is an active world of people with aphasia. There are the opportunities to reach out, make new friends and become involved. The choice is yours. You cannot help what happened to you. But you can chose how you react. While it may take some time before you are ready, we do encourage you to life live to the fullest with aphasia and not self-isolate.

One of ARC's active members is stroke survivor Avi Golden. He refuses to give up and continues to stay active. Before his stroke, Avi was a paramedic and about to start medical school. Avi was extremely active and loved many different outdoor sports like horseback riding, kayaking, sailing, bicycle riding and snowboarding.

When Avi was 33, he had a massive stroke that weakened his right side and resulted in aphasia. Avi didn't let his stroke hold him back. He started a group called New York Outdoor Disability that helps people with disabilities participate in outdoor sports. He also continues to volunteer as a paramedic and participates in a variety of plays. He advocates for people with aphasia and stays as active as possible. Inside, he is still the same driven and smart individual, and he hasn't let his stroke change who he is.

Like Avi, you will find adjusting to life with aphasia is challenging. You will have many hurdles to overcome. It will be frustrating when people assume that you are not intelligent just because you struggle to communicate.

But, like Avi, you can make goals for yourself to stay active. Volunteer, get outside, exercise, call friends and try to continue doing things you love to do. Therapy doesn't have to be the only opportunity you have to improve your language function. Life itself provides endless challenges of real world situations to improve your skills.

Set a goal today to find ways to connect with an online support group, an Aphasia Center in your area, a university that may have a clinic. Ask your speech therapist or family member to help you.

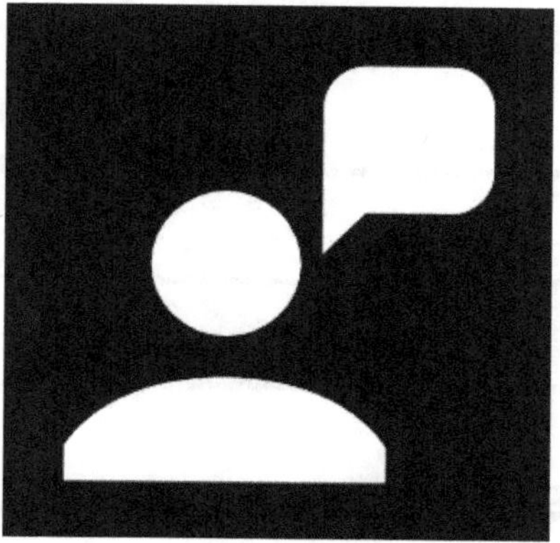

Self Evaluation

➢ **Who is in my circle of support?**

____

____

____

____

➢ **What are activities I can do today?**

____

____

____

____

➢ **What are activities I *want* to do even if I am not able to do it yet?**

____

____

____

____

➢ **What is my goal for today to help me connect?**

____

____

____

<table>
<tr><td>Other Notes:</td></tr>
<tr><td></td></tr>
<tr><td></td></tr>
<tr><td></td></tr>
<tr><td></td></tr>
<tr><td></td></tr>
</table>

> ➤ **What is Neuroplasticity?**

> ➤ **How Can I Help Neuroplasticity?**

> ➤ **How Does Rehabilitation work?**

What is Neuroplasticity?

There is good news! The brain has an amazing ability to change to promote recovery. Areas of the brain that survived can take on new functions. This is called **neuroplasticity**.

Aphasia is a result of damaged brain cells in the language center of your brain. The left hemisphere typically is the dominant hemisphere for both language comprehension and production. Broca's area, located in the left frontal lobe of the brain, controls language production while Wernicke's area lies on the left posterior temporal lobe of the brain and controls language comprehension. All strokes, no matter what kind, damage brain cells. The size and location of the lesion caused by your stroke or brain injury will determine what type of aphasia you have. You can refer to the image below to see where the Broca and Wernicke areas are.

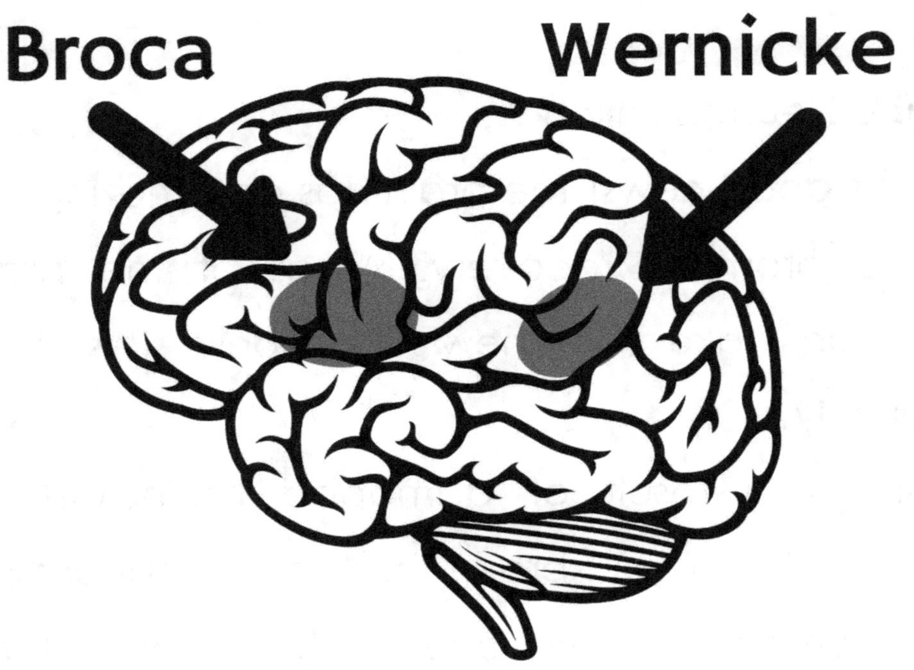

Language is a series of messages sent throughout the brain from one neuron to the next. When overcoming trauma, the human brain is remarkable and has the capability to reorganize areas of the brain and can even switch language center from one part of the brain to another. The brain can also build new neural connections to repair damaged areas. This is called neuroplasticity. Basically, the brain has the ability to repair and build new neural pathways after a stroke or brain injury that has damaged brain cells.

After a stroke or brain injury, the brain is able to repair itself at the neural level by growing new neurons. New neural pathways are formed when one axon grows new nerve endings to reconnect neurons that were severed as a result of damage from a stroke or brain injury.[xxx] In other words, new neural pathways are formed to reconnect areas of the brain. Because of neuroplasticity, continued recovery of both physical and language function is possible through rehabilitation.

Neuroplasticity: The Key to Rehabilitation

You just suffered a stroke or brain injury and may be feeling discouraged. But in the world of rehabilitation, strokes and brain injury recovery can be very promising. Neuroplasticity makes continued recovery possible. It will not be easy. Honestly, it is often a very slow process. It takes constantly challenging yourself to progress - and often you will not notice any improvement. **But keep working.** Recovery is a marathon - not a sprint - and many survivors report ongoing gains for months and years post stroke.

Unlike some progressive diseases (Parkinson's, Multiple Sclerosis or ALS), stroke survivors have the potential to improve. Neurogenesis is the growth of new brain cells and makes recovery of language and physical function possible.[xxxi] There are things you can do to help facilitate neurogenesis.

Aphasia Tip

When you wake up every morning, remind yourself, "My brain is repairing itself." Your positive self-talk matters.

recover and regain function. Use every available resource to help your brain recover and regain function.

> When David was recovering in the early years, Carol would whisper to him as he was falling asleep each night, "I am getting better. I will improve." It was very important that David believed he would get better. Without hope, why bother trying?

How Rehabilitation Works

We know that the brain has the capability to rewire itself through the power of neuroplasticity. This doesn't happen overnight and a balance of patient motivation, strong community support and rehabilitation all come together to make continued improvement possible.

How Does Challenging the Brain Help You Improve?

Strokes can cause weakness or paralysis on one side of the body either in an arm or a leg. With aphasia the brain has difficulty with word retrieval and sometimes speech can be slurred (dysarthria) or have motor planning difficulties (apraxia). Remember that with all of these challenges, initially the muscles and nerves in the legs, arms, tongue and face have not been directly damaged—it is the brain where the damage occurred. By **moving the impaired area** with assistance of a therapist and using muscles surrounding the weakened area you can stimulate the brain near the damaged area. **This stimulation can promote neurogenesis - repairing those pathways.**

Research studies have shown that even small repetitive exercises, such as moving your thumb back and forth for 15 minutes, can cause the brain to form new neural connections.[xxxii]Physical therapists utilize constraint-induced movement therapy for stroke survivors. This is a type of strategy that constrains the unaffected arm of a stroke survivor with hemiparesis, forcing them to use the arm that had been weakened by the stroke.[xxxiii]

The weak limb is isolated to complete daily tasks and tackle exercises, which produced great results in rehabilitation. This same concept has been carried over into language therapy for aphasia.

Aphasia is unique to stroke impairments because there is not any visible impairment. The neural pathways for word retrieval in the language center of the brain have been damaged. To translate the concept of small exercises for aphasia try repeating communication activities throughout the day that are easy for you. And, try to challenge yourself to do a little more. For example, you see the TV and you say, "TV." Then you might push yourself to say, "TV on." Then, "Turn TV on." Finally, "I will turn the TV on."

While talking out loud might not something you did a lot of before your stroke or injury, we encourage you to talk as much as you can.

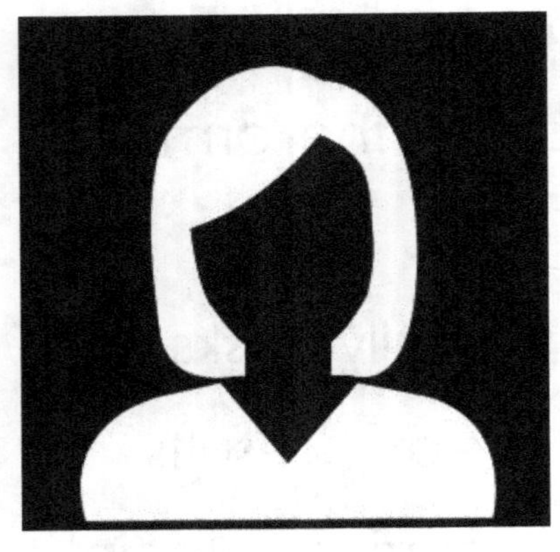

Ask your SLP

> *What are some repetition activities I can do?*
> *What other exercises or computer apps might help me?*

Even if you have speech therapy 5 times a week for an hour each time, that is less than 3% of the week that you spend in speech therapy.

For best results, you will want to start doing some of the exercises that you do in therapy during the day and make it part of your daily routine.

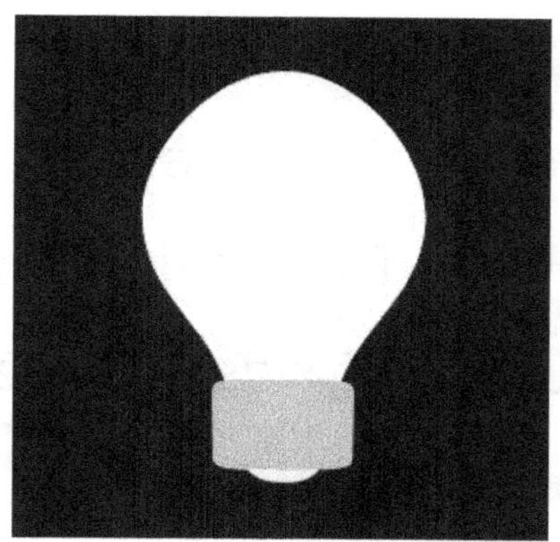

Aphasia Tips

Repetition is essential to improving both motor function and language function.[xxxiv]

> ➢ Start by trying to say aloud what you do throughout the day.

> ➢ Name items around your room as you use them if you are able.

> ➢ After a commercial on TV, say the name of the product that is for sale.

> ➢ Narrate what you do as you do it. "I'm picking up my hair brush. I'm moving it from the top of my head to the back of my head."

Even if you are only able to get one or two words out, it is the attempt that matters. The attempt stimulates the brain to begin the formation of new neural pathways.

It is important to stay active and communicate as much as possible using words or strategies.

Challenge yourself and even if something is frustrating, remember that a frustrating task is one that promotes the formation of new neural pathways.

David states in his book, *Brain Attack*, "Stroke survivors need to fight for recovery with determination and hope. It takes a long time to recover."

There are many resources available to help carry over therapy and make recovery part of your life, not just the hour or so you spend in speech therapy every week.

Motivation, family and community support, social interaction, and determination to challenge yourself to get better is the perfect mix for a strong recovery.

If you wanted to build your biceps, it would take consistent, daily effort with motivation and persistence, right? It you wanted to build you biceps but didn't commit to the work involved, you would not make progress.

If you want to improve your aphasia, it will take consistent, daily effort with motivation and persistence with repetition of activities. And a commitment to work involved to challenge yourself and promote recovery. It isn't easy. In fact, it is overwhelming and discouraging at times - but you need to keep moving forward. Set daily goals that are realistic for yourself and stick to your plan!

Self Evaluation

➤ **What repetition activities can I do today?**

____

____

____

➤ **What is my positive self-talk?**

____

____

➤ **What is easy for me?**

____

____

____

____

➤ **What is harder?**

____

____

____

> ## **Am I challenging myself with tasks throughout the day?**

____

____

____

Other Notes:

6

Speech & Language
THERAPY

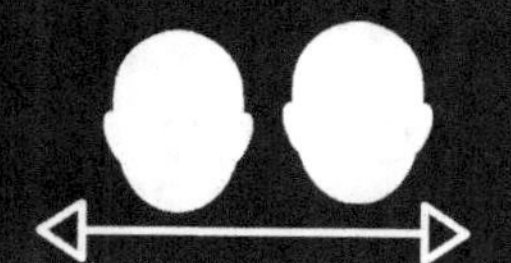

> ➢ Types of Aphasia Therapy and Treatments?

> ➢ What is Computer-based Therapy

> ➢ What is Constraint-induced Therapy?

> ➢ What is Melodic Intonation Therapy?

> ➢ What is Word Finding Treatment?

> ➢ What are Multi-Modal Treatments?

> ➢ What is Visual Action Treatment?

> ➢ What is Promoting Aphasia Communication Effectiveness (PACE)?

> ➢ What is Oral Reading for Language in Aphasia (ORLA?)

> ➢ What is Semantic Feature Analysis?

> ➢ What is Verb Network Strengthening Treatment (VneST)

> ➢ Can my Partner Help?

> ➢ What is the Life Participation Approach?

> ➢ What is Script Training?

> ➢ What are tDCS and rTMS?

Since no two cases of aphasia are exactly the same, there are many types of speech therapy approaches. Therapy builds on neuroplasticity by starting with language tasks that you are able to do and gradually increasing the difficulty level to improve your ability with harder tasks. This chapter will explain the common types of speech therapy techniques for aphasia. Your Speech-Language Pathologist can individualize your treatment and focus on goals that are the most important to you.

Aphasia Treatments

American Speech-Language-Hearing Association (**ASHA**) has recognized the therapies described in this chapter as potential treatments for aphasia. It is unlikely your therapist will use just one type of treatment. Ideally, your therapy will combine a variety of these approaches.[xxxv] It will be helpful to know what types of therapy are available.

Computer-based Therapy

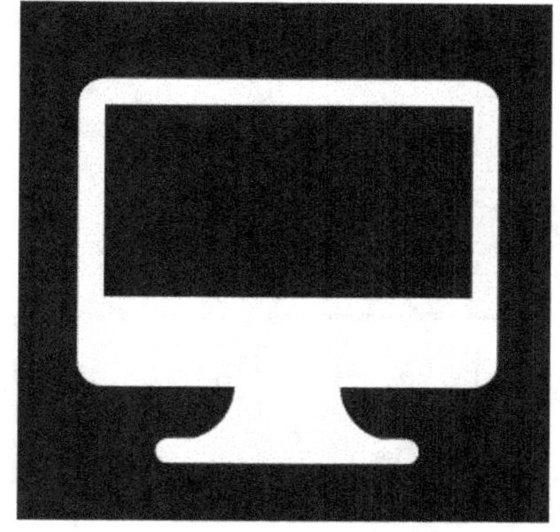

Computer software programs for aphasia allow for specific training on a language deficit. Computer based treatments are helpful to track progress and demonstrate improvement. Some of the benefits of computer based therapy include: flexibility, repetition, and the ability to personalize language exercises.[xxxvi] There are many options to choose from if you are looking for a computer based program to use. AphasiaSoftwareFinder.org provides a helpful list of available aphasia software.

Many people find that using apps designed by aphasia experts are an excellent way to challenge themselves with repetitive activities. One example Carol often recommends for patients in the hospital is Tactus Therapy's Alpha Topics. It includes a white board, alphabet, and yes/no. It can be adjusted in the settings to make it work best for you. Many apps have trial versions, so you can try before you purchase.

She shares, "David and I played a lot of Charades. Years later, as therapy apps and communication supports were developed, I so wished we had those tools too. Families today can benefit greatly from the technology available – to help reduce frustrations that can build up when communication breaks down."

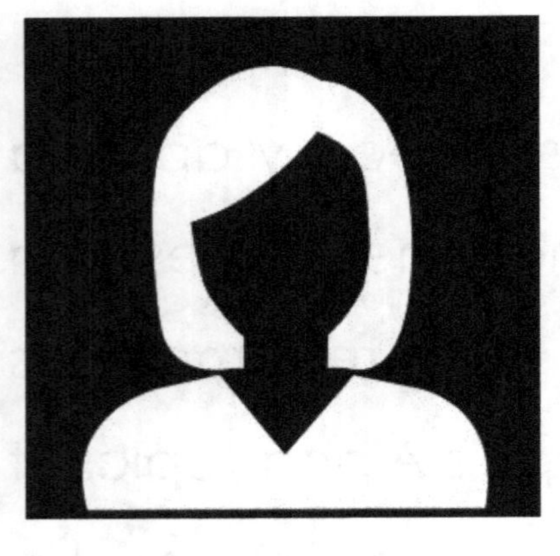

Ask your SLP

➢ *I'd like to try a computer software program for aphasia.*

➢ *What programs do you have?*

➢ *What programs do you recommend?*

Constraint Induced Language Therapy

Constraint induced language therapy, or CILT, is based on the concept that if you force yourself to use the mode of communication that is the hardest, you will make the most progress. CILT is typically an intensive program of up to 3 hours a day, 5 days a week. Your speech therapist will help with cues to initiate speech during communication tasks. CILT discourages use of aphasia compensatory strategies such as gestures or writing and focuses solely on verbal responses. CILT takes advantage of neuroplasticity to structure tasks that facilitate the formation of new neural connections in the language centers of the brain.

Constraint induced therapy that incorporates gradual steps up to difficult tasks, like describing with multiple adjectives, has been shown to have excellent results for individuals who were told they had already reached their maximum post-stroke potential.[xxxvii] The basis of constraint induced therapy for aphasia is to incorporate the most difficult communication tasks into therapy and everyday life to achieve the highest levels of expressive language communication abilities. Challenging yourself to try harder things at small increments is key.

Melodic Intonation Therapy

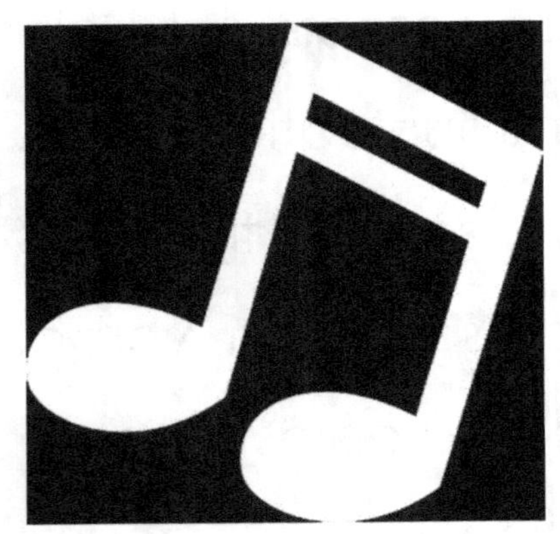

Melodic Intonation Therapy (MIT) utilizes rhythm and melody to improve expressive language function. The right hemisphere of the brain controls our ability to listen to and produce music. Most people who have aphasia have sustained damage to the left hemisphere of the brain. Melodic Intonation Therapy recruits the right hemisphere using music to help with language tasks.

MIT therapy is usually presented in four stages. In the first stage, the therapist and patient will hum a phrase from a familiar song. For the second phrase, the patient and therapist will sing the words together. Next, the person with aphasia will sing the phrase independently. In the fourth and final stage, the person with aphasia may be able to speak the phrase.[xxxviii] During Melodic Intonation Therapy, SLPs sometimes incorporate melody into conversations and have a person with aphasia participate in a conversation by singing the answers to questions.

Finger tapping is also utilized to help facilitate rhythmic speech and recruit additional regions of the brain to help with expressive language. [xxxix] ARC's Virtual Connections sometimes offers music sessions including Melodic Intonation sessions online.

Word Finding Treatment

Word finding difficulty, or anomia, is often a symptom of aphasia. Most types of aphasia have some degree of anomia associated with it. Speech-Language Pathologists will use cues to help a person with aphasia say a specific word.

Semantic cues are verbal prompts related to the meaning of the word. For example, if you are trying to say *bed*, your SLP may cue you by saying "sleep", "lie down in it", or "king-sized."

The SLP may also use phonemic cues, which are the initial sounds of the word you want to say. For example, if you are trying to name a photograph of a shoe, your SLP would make the sound "sh" to help you retrieve the word. If you are stuck on the word "dog", the prompt "It's raining cats and _____" may help you say dog. Often, these cues with the flow of a sentence and the first sound, may help you get the word out. Your SLP may also use carrier phrases to decrease anomia.

Gesture cues are also helpful with word finding tasks. Using your hand to pretend to use an object, triggers other areas of your brain to help retrieve the desired word.

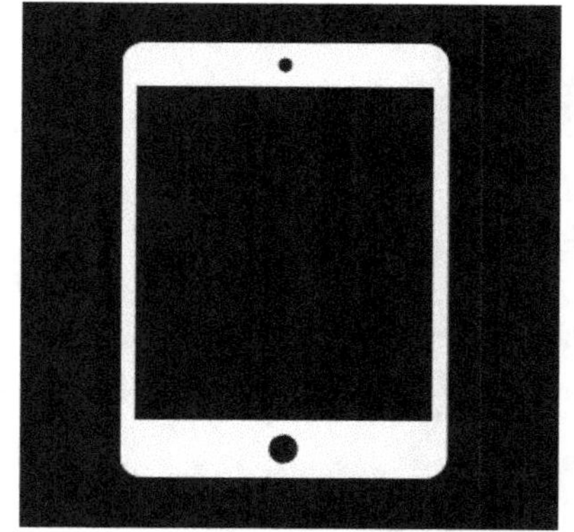

Multimodal Treatment, AAC

Multimodal treatment focuses on using alternative modes of communication. Augmentative and Alternative Communication (AAC) is an example of an alternative mode of communication. AAC devices can be basic picture images on a communication board or a complex computer device designed to help an individual with aphasia communicate. There is also software available for your tablet that can function as an AAC device. Individuals with very limited expressive language function can benefit greatly from using an AAC device.

Your SLP can help you pick an AAC device that best suits your needs. These devices are often covered by insurance for those with aphasia and you may qualify for a free trial.

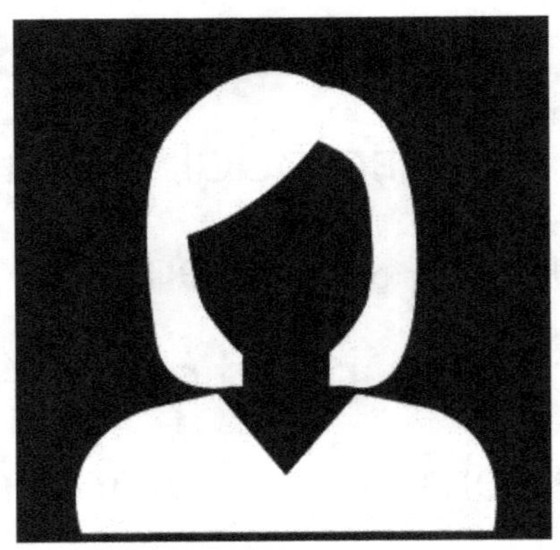

Ask your SLP

> *I am interested in trying an AAC device*

Carol shares: "We have discovered that not all speech therapists are trained in AAC devices as this is a specialty focus." If you want to see what a device looks like or may be capable of to support your independence, click here: aphasia.com "If you want to talk to a therapist who specializes in AAC devices, this company will be able to provide you with some expert guidance."

While some believe that a "device" to support communication is going to diminish your skills, it often improves your skills as it supports your independence and peace of mind, resulting in more language attempts, not less.

Just like a wheelchair is given to a person with the hope they may not need it later, a device may be given to you with the hope you eventually will not need it.

> Carol adds, "The peace of mind for the person with aphasia and the family members is incredible. As a caregiver, knowing my loved one can navigate the world or an ER visit independently without my being there –gives both of us peace of mind. There is a learning curve with set up – but in the long run – this is a wonderful option for those with aphasia."

Visual Action Therapy

Visual Action Therapy is a treatment approach used with individuals with global aphasia. This approach teaches individuals with global aphasia to communicate using hand and arm gestures.[xl] The Visual Action Therapy treatment approach is appropriate for individuals with severe expressive and comprehension deficits. Visual Action Therapy uses real objects, line drawings of objects and pictures of people using objects. This therapy approach combines pointing to objects and gesturing the function of objects to improve expressive and receptive language function.[xli]

Promoting Aphasia Communication Effectiveness (PACE)

This type of therapy can be tried at home. You will need photographs of functional objects or index cards with the names of objects written on them. As the items become easier for you, try using verbs or picture scenes.

For this type of exercise, select a photograph of an item and then you and a partner will take turns trying to guess what the photo is. It is similar to the game "20 questions" but instead of asking and answering yes or no questions, ask some that require a description for an answer—open-ended questions. Questions such as "Where can you find it?", "What do you use it for?", "Who uses it?" and "When do you use it?" are ideal because they require a descriptive answer. PACE encourages a person with aphasia to communicate any way possible by drawing, writing, gesturing, and describing. [xlii] Your partner or a volunteer can help as well by using the cuing technique. If the photo was a pair of socks and you struggled with the word, your loved one could gesture as though putting on socks, saying, " I am putting on my shoes and s____." (They give you the first sound of the word.) Your local office supply store or teacher store often has flashcards that may be helpful. We suggest you also look at ESL suppliers (English as a Second Language) as they flashcards may be more adult oriented.

Oral Reading for Language in Aphasia (ORLA)

ORLA therapy is also something you can do at home on your own or with a family member or friend. If your reading aloud skills are strong, this can be an easy way to carry over therapy at home. With ORLA, the person with aphasia reads sentences aloud, first in unison with a partner and then independently. Try pacing yourself with your finger as you point to each word and keep a steady rhythm as you read. Repeating the same sentences several times is recommended. As you improve, you can move on to reading paragraphs and passages aloud. Research has shown that practicing reading aloud with a partner and then independently can carry over to improved expressive language skills.[xliii] Lingraphica offers many free educational resources on their website. To learn more about ORLA go here:

http://www.aphasia.com/aphasia-resource-library/aphasia-treatments/orla/.

> Carol found that David did much better with larger print books. Often, people with aphasia find that materials in the ESL (English as a Second Language) section of a library to be helpful as they are designed for adults with limited language.

Semantic Feature Analysis

Semantic Feature Analysis treatment is a type of treatment that focuses on improving word retrieval. Semantic features are different properties about an item that describe its meaning. The semantic features of the word girl include young, human and female. For this treatment approach, you can either use a photo or the word and describe different characteristics about the word. For example, after seeing a photo of a toaster, you would be cued to answer questions about the features. For example: What room would you find this? (kitchen); What is it used for? (toast bread); What meal is it used for most? (breakfast). [xliv]

You can find these exercises and much more in the *Speech Therapy Aphasia Rehabilitation Workbook I* by this book's co-author, Amanda P. Anderson.

Verb Network Strengthening Treatment (VNeST)

This treatment approach targets verbs to promote word retrieval at the sentence level. For example, the person with aphasia is given a verb (e.g., *cook)* and is asked to answer "who cooks what?"[xlv] It can eventually target written skills depending on the patient's severity level. The person with aphasia can write multiple subject-verb-object sentences for each verb. (eg., The chef cooks filet mignon, She cooks bacon, I cook dessert etc.).

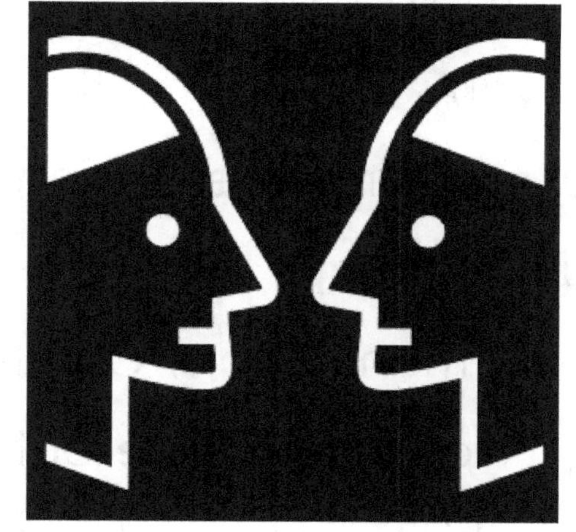

Partner Approaches

Partner approaches have the Speech-Language Pathologist work together with the person with aphasia and somebody they have the most interaction with, such as a spouse or children. Conversational Coaching Therapy concentrates on communication between you and your most frequent conversational partner. Supported Communication Intervention therapy involves an SLP helping a person with aphasia and a family member communicate together.

Speech Therapy for aphasia can be highly individualized. You can work on communication goals that are most important to you. Some people with aphasia are able to have a conversation with their SLP after they have worked together, but they continue to struggle when they try to speak to family members.

You can also have your speech therapist work with you and your family members so you can practice communication goals at home. You can practice talking with your spouse or family member during therapy.

While David continued in therapy for many years, Carol shared this story. "I thought I was an excellent communication partner. I'd read everything I could about aphasia. Then, one day the SLP worked with David behind a two-way mirror so I could observe. I was amazed at his capabilities with her! It wasn't until I actually saw the techniques in action that I truly became a better communication partner."

Ask your SLP:

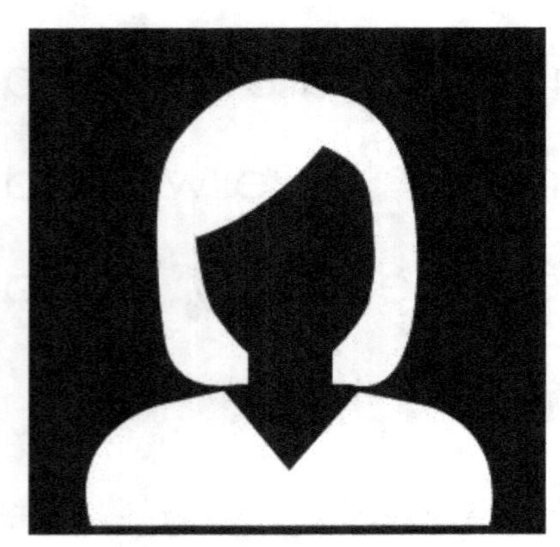

> *I want to practice communicating with my spouse/family/friend.*

> *Please show my family members how to work on my therapy goals with me.*

Life Participation Approach

Aphasia researchers, clinicians and people with aphasia have determined that the most successful approach to rehabilitation focuses on increasing participation in communication activities meaningful to the person with aphasia.[xlvi] Life Participation Approach to Aphasia (LPAA) concentrates on real life communication goals as a part of therapy. The focus of the Life Participation Approach to Aphasia is to help a person with aphasia participate in communication situations where they may need support. Goals are made based on community interaction and the level of support an individual wants to participate in desired activities. Therapy can focus on overcoming communication obstacles by treating both the person with aphasia and the people they interact with the most.

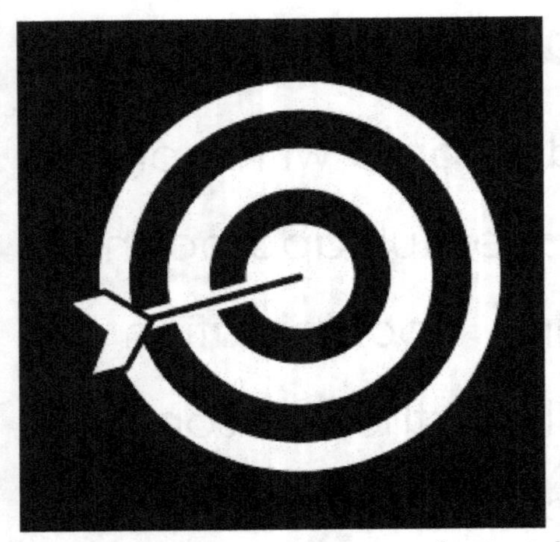

Life Participation Approach is a model of therapy that embraces **goals** to reduce barriers in day-to-day communication. Types of goals for this approach range from communicating with family to challenges associated with returning to work, depending on which area requires the most focus.

Speech-Language Pathologists work to make a person's environment more "aphasia-friendly." This model of therapy not only focuses on the person with aphasia but others who are indirectly affected by aphasia, like family members, friends, colleagues, and service providers. It is a patient-centered philosophy that gives priority to real life situations.

The American Stroke Association provides a list of aphasia centers that integrate LPAA into their mission. You can find this list in the Appendix.

Script Training

Script Training is a type of therapy that you can try at home. Scripts can be used with many types of aphasia and are most successful when they are practiced over and over. Repetition of a script leads to carryover of communication skills. Your SLP can help create a script you can practice at home with a partner.

Pick something you are interested in and something that is a real life situation such as: calling to order a pizza, making a doctor's appointment, talking about the birth of a child or a favorite vacation destination. The most successful scripts are fun and personally meaningful. Ideal scripts are about 8 to 15 sentences long and have around 8 turn-taking sets.[xlvii]

Scripts can be monologues where somebody is the only speaker or dialogues that require a partner to ask and answer questions.

Practice short scripts such as:

1. "Hello. My name is ___.

   I had a stroke."

2. "Hello. My name is _________.

   I had a stroke _____ years ago."

3. "Hello. My name is ________. I had a stroke.

      Please be patient.

4. Hello. My name is ________.

   My favorite pastime is: _______.

Next you can try a more challenging two-person dialogue script such as this one:

Script: Ordering a Pizza

   Thanks for calling Pappy's Pizza. Can I help you?

   You: Yes, I'd like to order a large pizza.

   Would you like any toppings?

   You: Yes, pepperoni and sausage.

   Would you like any side items?

   You: Yes, I'd like an order of breadsticks with extra

   dipping sauce.

   Anything else?

   You: Yes, I'd like a 2-liter bottle of Sprite

   What is your address?

   You: (Say your address)

What time would you like the pizza delivered?

You: Right away please.

How would you like to pay?

You: Cash.

Thank you for your order. It should arrive in 45 minutes.

You: Great! Thank you.

If you are able, you could practice reading the script over and over until you have memorized it and do not need the written cues. Make scripts that are real life situations so they can carry over into your everyday communication. If you are unable to read, you might have a loved one record a video or audio, so you can listen and practice.

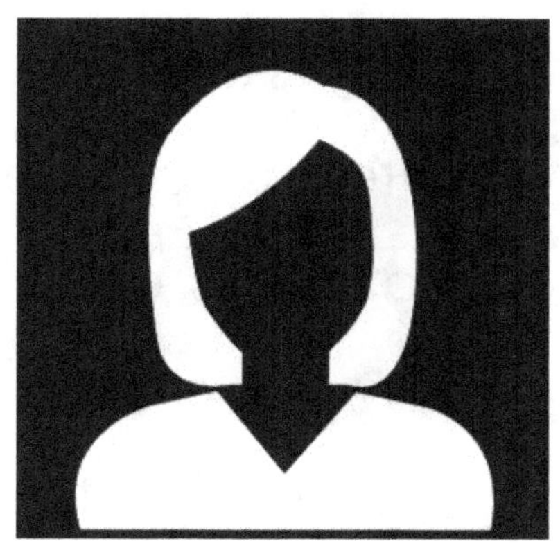

Ask your SLP

➢ *Please help me make a script that I can practice at home.*

tDCS and rTMS

Transcranial Direct Current Stimulation (tDCS) and Repetitive Transcranial Magnetic Stimulation (rTMS) are non-invasive forms of brain stimulation. The biggest difference is that tDCS is a small headgear that uses a battery and TMS is usually powered by electricity on the wall and uses a coil placed over your head.

They have been in use since the 1980s to help treat depression but recently have been utilized in aphasia treatment. As of 2019, ASHA's systematic review of the effectiveness of tDCS concluded, "There was no evidence of an effect of tDCS for improving functional communication in adults with aphasia. However, there was limited evidence that tDCS improved naming skills post-intervention and at follow up."[xlviii] Despite limited evidence to improve naming skills in aphasia, these treatments could have potential positive benefits.

To date, there are multiple clinical trials investigating the efficacy of both tDCS and rTMS in aphasia treatment.

Check clinicaltrials.gov/ for studies that may be recruiting participants near you.

We are not recommending this or any treatments. We are sharing it for anyone that may hear about this treatment and have an interest. As with many treatments, it may indeed be contraindicated. For example, while hyperbaric oxygen treatment is somewhat controversial, many try it. However, David's doctor has strictly forbidden it due to the cause of his stroke. As with any treatment, consult with your health professional for guidance.

Other Aphasia Treatments

Some people with aphasia have difficulty with specific language tasks. There are specialized aphasia therapy programs to isolate the area where a person with aphasia is having trouble. For example, Reading Treatment, Writing Treatment, Syntax Treatment, Treatment of Underlying Forms and Verb Network Strengthening Treatment are all specialized aphasia therapy techniques.[xlix] To read more about these specific therapies and evidence-based research showing the data from clinical studies, visit asha.org

Remember that **you** are in charge of your rehabilitation. If you feel that you want to vary the challenge or make a change with a new therapist, it is up to you to voice these goals and desires. It need not be a reflection on your current therapist. Sometimes, a change is fresh and exciting—and we all tend to get bored if there are no changes in our lives. Over the course of David's years in speech therapy, he had over 25 different therapists. "Each one had different techniques. But if they weren't committed and challenging me, I changed therapists."

Not every speech therapist is an aphasia specialist. Some specialize in pediatrics. Others are experts in swallowing disorders. Some specialize in communication devices. Your recovery team is very important, so a good aphasia therapist is important. If there is not an aphasia specialist in your area that fits your needs, you might consider tele-therapy.

Carol adds, "I think it is better to get quality effective treatment based on research and experience than quantity of treatment by someone who may have very limited experience in treating aphasia."

Your SLP will likely use a combination of these techniques to best meet your needs. If you continue to do the same exercises over and over, and you haven't seen any improvement outside of therapy, it is okay to ask your SLP to modify your treatment plan.

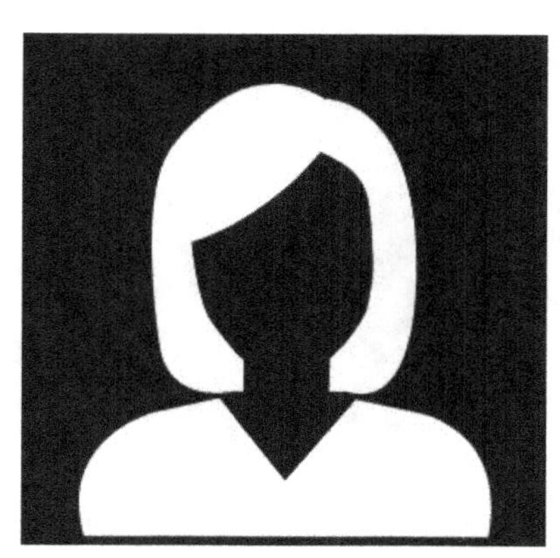

Ask your SLP:

> ***Can we try another approach to therapy?***

> ***I am interested in including my family in therapy.***

> ***I'm getting frustrated with our current exercises; can we try something else?***

> ***I feel successful when I read aloud. Can we work that into therapy?***

> ***I would like to practice using my tablet apps in therapy.***

> ***I would like to give Melodic Intonation Therapy a try.***

➢ **Can we set goals of what I am interested in?**

➢ **I want to learn to Zoom (or other options).**

➢ **Can you connect me to Facebook so I can meet others?**

➢ **Can you recommend a program of things I can do in my free time?**

Self Evaluation

➢ **What are my therapy goals?**

____

____

____

____

➢ **What therapy or therapies are easy for me?**

____

____

____

> **What therapy or therapies are hard for me?**

____

____

____

____

> **What questions do I have for my SLP?**

____

____

____

____

> **What are my interests?**

____

____

____

____

➢ **What activities do I want to get back to in the next month? In the next year?**

____

____

____

➢ **What treatment options do I want to consider?**

____

____

____

➢ **Is my therapist a good fit for me and my goals?**

____

____

____

7

Tools You Can Use
TECHNOLOGY

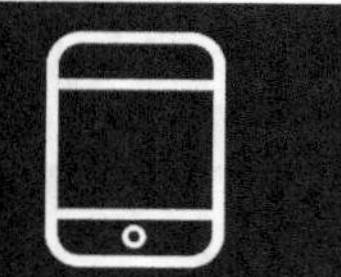

> **What Technology Can Help People With Aphasia?**

> **What Are Some Apps That Can Help?**

In this age of tablets (e.g. iPads) and smartphones, there are many helpful programs for aphasia. Technology can be utilized for assisting with communication. Speech therapy computer software or tablet applications for aphasia can be used on your own or with a Speech-Language Pathologist. Including technology in your rehabilitation is also a helpful way to maximize your recovery potential.

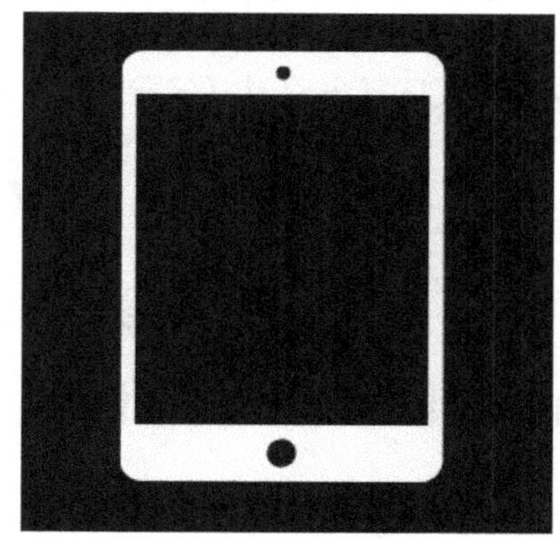

Tablets

If you used a tablet before aphasia, continue to use what you are familiar with if it works for you. If you've never used a tablet before, it may be worth the investment to purchase one. Many

SLPS recommend purchasing an iPad, to have access to the widest variety of programs (or *apps,* as they're often called). To save money, you could purchase a used or refurbished iPad, but make sure that it is compatible with the latest software you plan on using for your rehabilitation.

Sometimes, tools that were easy to use before your aphasia, may prove more difficult now. Ask your SLP if it is a good option for you at this time.

Kindle devices are more affordable and have many options for aphasia apps. You can search for aphasia apps on the amazon website. Search for 'aphasia' and click the arrow next to the search bar to select apps for Androids. This will show you what is available. You can ask ARC members on Facebook for feedback about a particular app. With thousands of members, they are often a great resource to ask when you have a question.

If you do not have access to a computer, getting a tablet will function as both a device that can access the internet, a supportive communication tool, and provide access to apps for speech therapy exercises.

David used technology apps to supplement his therapy and later continued when insurance no longer covered his treatment.

Social Media: Facebook

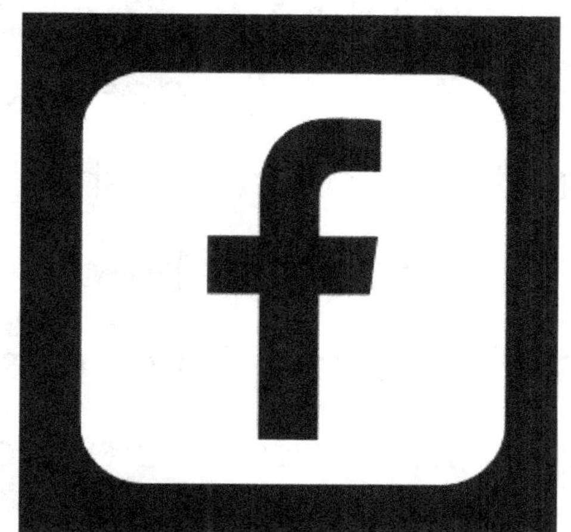

Aphasia Recovery Connection has a private Facebook group and a public page that are great resources and offer peer support within a virtual community. ARC members on Facebook enjoy having a place where they can communicate and practice their skills such as reading, writing and posting videos. Spelling doesn't matter. It is a group who understands the challenges you are now faced with. ARC's Facebook group also offers the opportunity to receive support as well as socializing with other people with aphasia.

We encourage you to join the group to meet other families that are also navigating this aphasia journey. Appendix D explains how to create a Facebook account.

There are multiple groups on Facebook that are beneficial for stroke survivors. ARC has groups for caregivers as well called ARC Care Partners. There are groups for young stroke survivors and their family members. (ARC: Kids with Aphasia) Facebook can be a wonderful resource to find support from others who are dealing with similar issues.

The Speech Therapy Aphasia Rehabilitation (STAR) group on Facebook provides free therapy exercises for people with aphasia. There, you can post questions to co-author Amanda, who is a speech therapist. Find her workbooks on Amazon.

APPS

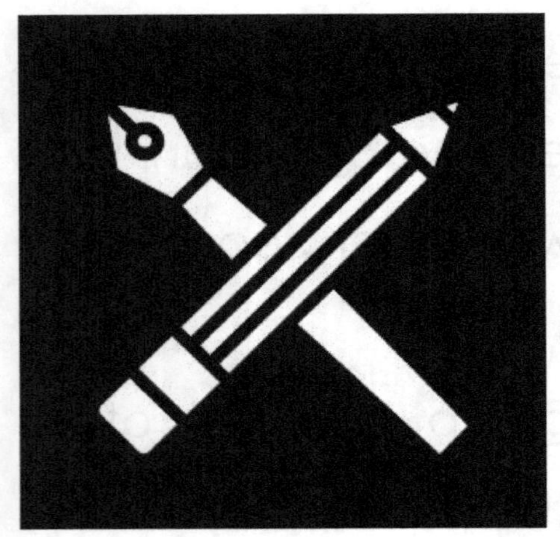

An app (short for application) is something you can download onto either a smartphone or tablet like an iPad or Kindle device. There are many free apps that you can use on your mobile device of choice.

If you search for "flash cards", lots of free options with many naming categories will come up. You can use basic flash cards to work on word retrieval skills. Try to select one where you can mute the word. It might be helpful at first to have the app say the name of the object with you initially and, as you improve, you can mute the word. You can also search for "aphasia" for apps with more appropriate exercises for aphasia.

Some fun examples include the app "Heads Up" that Ellen DeGeneres plays on her show requires you to describe the word that somebody holds up above their head, and they have to guess what it is. This is an excellent game to work on descriptive language skills that promotes the formation of new neural pathways. "Heads Up" also comes in a board game edition. The game "Catch Phrase" is also a great game for building descriptive language skills. ARC's Virtual Connections also hosts video chats about new and helpful apps for aphasia.

Here are some examples. While it may be tempting to start to upload or purchase many, we recommend you start with the appropriate one and master it rather than overwhelm yourself with too many apps.

Tactus Therapy offers a free PDF that is perfect to print out to help you review some of the options and it will help understand the activities and supports apps can offers. Find out more at this web address: tactustherapy.com/using-apps-treat-severe-aphasia/

Here is a list of Apps we have found helpful.

App List

Asking TherAppy

Locabulary Lite

Word Stack

Chain of Thought

Constant Therapy

Tactus Therapy Apps

Alicom

Sonoflex Lite

White Board

Make Change

Dollar and Cents

Words with Friends

Just Say It

Taboo

Oxford Picture Dictionary

Small Talk (scripts)

Pictello (scripts)

iConverse (scripts)

Video Assisted Speech Technology VASTtx

Some of the apps are free and some of them cost a few dollars. Therapy applications and software with a wide variety of exercises and goals can cost somewhat more. Keep in mind that some of those apps are excellent products and they often cost less than a speech therapy session if you were to pay out of pocket.

On aphasiarecoveryconnection.org you can find recommendations for current technology to help you communicate. Several other websites list apps and software for aphasia. Here are a few of them:

Aphasiasoftwarefinder.org

Tactustherapy.com

Constant Therapy

Amyspeechlanguagetherapy.com/

Augmentative and Alternative Communication (AAC)

Before smartphones and tablets, Augmentative and Alternative Communication (AAC) devices used to be bulky and awkward. Now there are some apps that you can download onto a device like an iPhone or iPad and use it to help you communicate. Earlier AAC devices stuck out and drew attention to the user. Today, almost everyone carries a smartphone or tablet and it isn't unusual to see somebody using one.

There are companies that offer a variety of AAC devices. These are handheld speech-generating devices. They also provide a variety of apps for speech therapy exercises as well as AAC on the go. Their website, aphasia.com, offers a wealth of information about their products and how to get help with funding.

Some apps function as AAC devices. The app *YesNo* provides two buttons for yes/no that you can customize with your own voice. The apps *Scene Speak*, and *Scene and Heard* are communication boards with voice output.[l] There are apps that function as complete AAC devices such as *MyVoice*, *Proloquo2Go* and *TalkTablet*. The full-functioning AAC apps range in price from $80 to around $200.[li]

As you compare, keep in mind that some are "one-time" purchases with free updates. Other companies may charge monthly fees that can add up to hundreds of dollars over time, but may be your preference. It is up to you, your family, your speech therapist, and your budget. But, we do suggest that you do not go out and buy several. That can be overwhelming. Make the right pick for you, find success and then build your app library over time. There is no rush!

Software

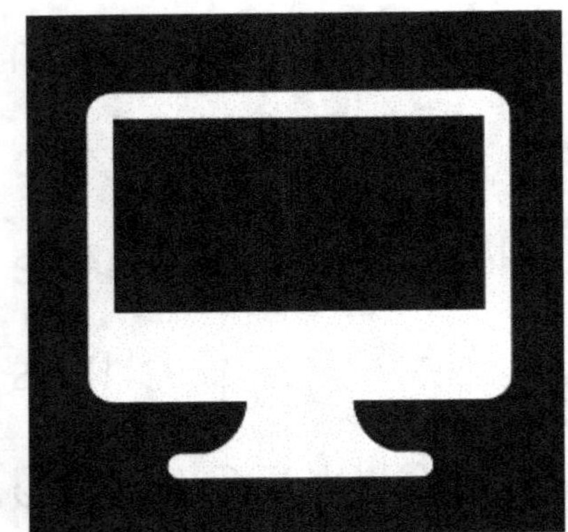

Software is similar to an app and can even be the same program, but it is something that you use on your computer or laptop. There is software available for people with aphasia. The Rehabilitation Institute of Chicago has aphasia script software programs using the script therapy technique. To view their software product go to:

ricaphasiascripts.contentshelf.com

NOTE: These are compatible only with PC not Macs or iOS devices like iPad, iPhone.

AphasiaSoftwareFinder.org has a nice aphasia-friendly list of aphasia software with a comparison table. Software programs can be an excellent way to continue speech therapy when benefits have expired, but also as a way to supplement active therapy.

eWriters

For people with aphasia who have strong writing skills or who need written cues to improve comprehension, an eWriter is an excellent option. eWriters are inexpensive (under $50) electronic notepads that you can clear with the touch of a button. Some models allow you to save your image. An eWriter doesn't require paper and pencils and the stylus (pen) clips onto the board, making it aphasia-friendly. This is a nice device to aid with communication for people with aphasia. One of the most widely available (and a favorite) is called the Boogie Board and available at places like Walmart or Amazon.

Other Technology

Kindle books are ones that you can read either on a computer, a smartphone, or tablet. You can "carry" multiple books on your tablet, which is aphasia-friendly, especially for people with right hand weakness. You can change the font size with digital books, which can help improve comprehension for some people with aphasia. Kindle books are relatively inexpensive compared to printed versions. You can also purchase aphasia workbooks for Kindle such as the first expressive language Speech Therapy Aphasia Rehabilitation STAR Workbook.

You can take advantage of tools that automatically come with your smartphone or tablet. The voice dictation on your smartphone can be a useful exercise. Turn it on and try reading or saying a sentence in a very clear rhythmic style. These voice dictation programs have difficulty perfectly recognizing what people without aphasia say, so it is sometimes quite a challenge, but will force you to speak in a slow rhythmic tone, which can help with expressive language function.

Phone conversations can be difficult for someone with aphasia. The computer program Zoom is a great way to make video calls. Video calls can help people with aphasia communicate much better over long distances. Video chats allow for the use of facial expressions, gestures, photographs, and nods to help you communicate much better with people than you could over the telephone. If you use iPhone or iPad or Mac computer Facetime is a free app already on your device that allows you to make video calls. And, the ARC Facebook Group has also expanded to use Messenger Rooms video conferencing.

Technology and Therapy

If working on a computer or tablet is difficult for you, it is a perfect goal for speech therapy or occupational therapy. Occupational therapy can focus on some of the fine motor challenges involved in manipulating a tablet or computer. Working with technology be a wonderful skill that will help you with your communication once your therapy insurance benefits have run out.

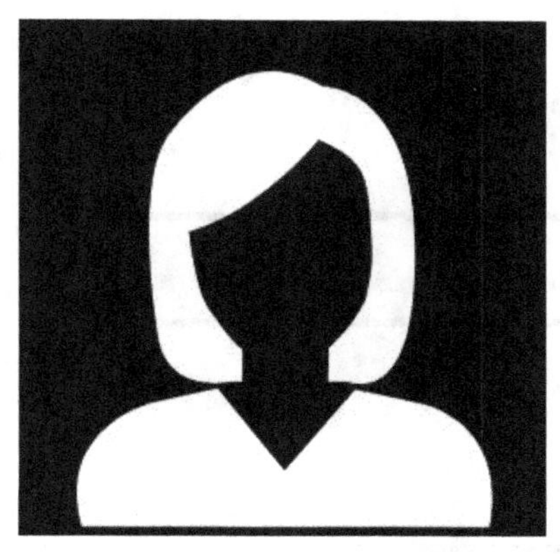

Ask your SLP

> *I'd like to make working on my tablet a goal for therapy.*
> *I want to learn how to use Facebook in therapy.*
> *I'd like to practice writing emails.*
> *I'd like to learn how to post a question on the ARC Facebook Group.*
> *I would like to practice making a video call or Facetime on my phone.*

> *I want to learn how to video-conference, like on Zoom to chat with others or my grandchildren.*

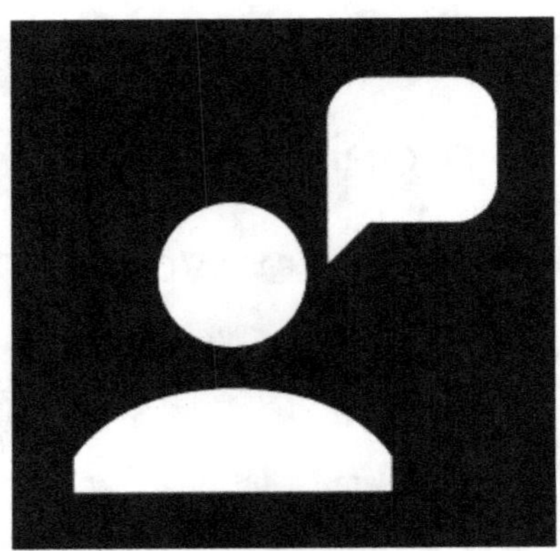

Self-evaluation

> **What technology am I interested in using?**

____

____

> **What technology do I own?**

____

____

> **Which technology is easy for me now? Which is hard?**

____

____

> **How Can I Cope With Aphasia?**

> **Is Depression Common?**

> **What Other Emotional Changes Can There Be?**

> **How Can I Stay Motivated?**

> **Is There Really Hope?**

Aphasia can cause an upheaval in every aspect of your life from career to relationships. Many people think aphasia is "just" a language disorder. The reality is - language affects jobs, relationships, sense of self, and peace of mind.

You are not alone. Over two million people in the United States have aphasia. David and Carol started the nonprofit Aphasia Recovery Connection because they know firsthand how hard it is.

ARC's main mission is to help end the isolation of aphasia as they help others navigate this bumpy road to recovery. Aphasia is extremely frustrating and often it is hard to find people, even health professionals, who are well versed in aphasia. People living with aphasia will tell you that having a support network like ARC can be a lifeline with their groups on Facebook.

Hope and motivation are your friends, isolation and despair are your enemies. Even so, it is still okay to cry, scream, or get angry. Feelings are real - and it is often helpful to express them rather than bury them.

Carol shares, "I know this is difficult. I lived this nightmare myself and know the feeling of being so very afraid and full of grief as a caregiver. I can only imagine how difficult it is for you. I know it is hard...and you must hang on to hope. Things do improve. However, it is often a very slow process."

Aphasia can be one of the most difficult challenges to cope with because of the lack of ability to communicate. Multiple studies have found that aphasia has a significant negative impact on quality of life.[lii] Communication is how we vent, how we feel better. When you get in a fight, you talk things out to make amends. When you are afraid, you talk about what is bothering you. When you are depressed, you talk to somebody about what is weighing on you. Aphasia robs you of these outlets.

One study showed that when compared to 75 other diseases and health conditions, aphasia had the biggest negative impact on health related quality of life on those living in long-term care.[liii] It is for that reason that ARC's mission focuses on the psychosocial aspects of your recovery, which is also very therapeutic and will challenge your language skills at the same time.

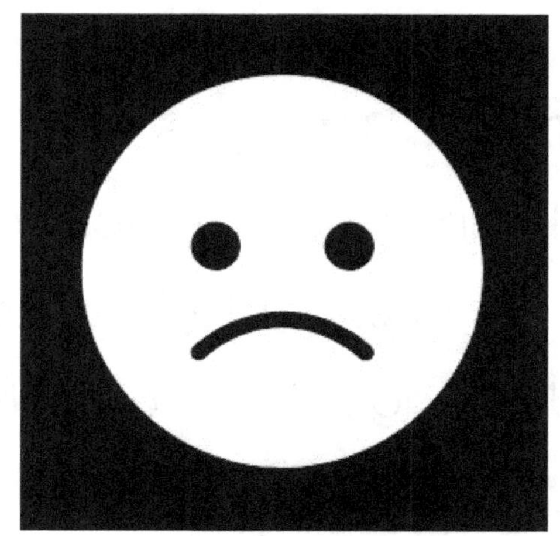

Depression

With so much to cope with, it is not surprising that as many as 62% of people with aphasia are clinically depressed one year after their stroke.[liv] Up to 33% of people with aphasia have major depression, at the one-year mark after their initial diagnosis.[lv] Stroke survivors may experience major depression, which results from a chemical imbalance in the brain[lvi] or as a result of such a tremendous life change.

A psychiatrist is a type of doctor can evaluate and determine if you would benefit from antidepressant medication or other treatment People with aphasia experience a great loss of their former abilities and go through a period of grief.[lvii] It is understandable to mourn. There is some controversy whether or not people experiencing grief go through set standard stages. [lviii] Remember, your journey of acceptance and coping is as unique as you and your aphasia.[lix]

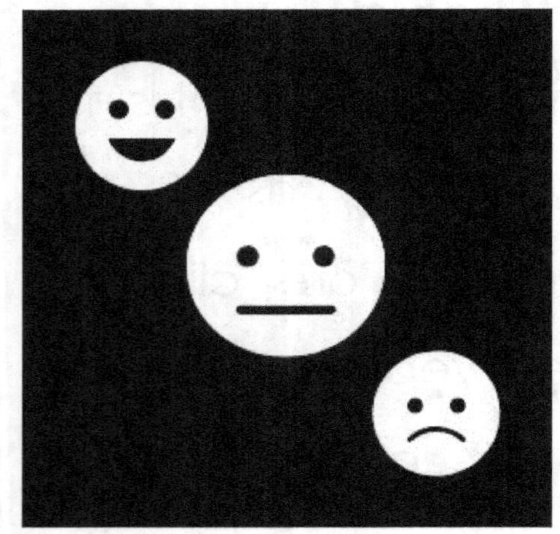

Emotional Changes

Stroke and brain injury survivors may experience unexpected and exaggerated changes in mood, which is called emotional lability.

You may find yourself crying for no apparent reason or laughing uncontrollably. Your stroke or brain injury may have damaged the part of your brain that regulates and controls emotions.[lx] It is important for family and friends to understand.

Changes in mood may result in increased irritability, anger or intense sadness. Sometimes the strong emotions such as crying or laughing are not related to how you are feeling inside. [lxi] Some stroke survivors have difficulty understanding their own emotions. The part of your brain that is able to pick up on others facial expressions and their emotions may have been damaged by your stroke or brain injury.

There is a condition called pseudobular affect than is not the same as depression, however people may cry for no reasons. This is a treatable condition and you should discuss this with your doctor if you feel you are crying or laughing for no reason.

Finding yourself struggling to process your emotions, and having difficulty picking up on subtleties of others' emotions is something that you can work on in speech therapy. Sometimes, just changing your activity helps. But we do know that mood disorders can hold back your recovery - so discussing these with your doctor may be key to optimizing your recovery and well-being[lxii].

Resources

For individuals with aphasia suffering from depression, traditional talk therapy may not be an effective option as most therapists are not training in aphasia and your own limited ability to express your feelings. Seek out support groups, either on Facebook or in your community. The National Aphasia Association has a search page to help you find support groups for aphasia in your area.

Visit National Aphasia Association (aphasia.org/sites_category/support-groups/) OR National Stroke Association (www.stroke.org/en/stroke-support-group-finder) to find a group in your area.

You may want to seek out the help of a psychiatrist. You can bring a friend or family member with you to help express what you are feeling. You can also ask your speech therapist to help you write down your concerns before you meet with a psychiatrist. The key is to recognize it and take action and address it early on. Remember, it is a common reaction and getting help is actually addressing the issue and empowering you to take an active role in your recovery.

Survivor David Dow shares with ARC members a tip to stay positive: "I know it is very difficult to be motivated and active during your recovery.

Don't be a couch potato. It is very easy for me and many people to sit on the couch and watch TV and not care about the world around you. It is very important to get out and keep moving and keep your brain active every day."

MotivationT

Try to push yourself to stay active and involved. If you you are able to do even if it takes longer.

If you are blessed with supportive people in your life, try not to let them do too much for you. Work hard to do the things you are able to do.

Carol shares a story where she learned more about David's desire to be more independent. "I found it difficult to leave David alone for any length of time as he needed help for almost everything, or so I thought. After a rare outing, my husband and I returned home to find a basket of cookies on the kitchen table. Hmm, someone must have dropped by for a visit. I wondered who had come by while we were out. David's aphasia made it impossible to just ask him, *Who brought the cookies?* Although he would know the answer, his stroke left him unable to speak. We relied on yes-or-no questions or used gestures to communicate.

I began my usual questioning. "Was it Sue?" No, David shook his head, looking annoyed.

I remembered that the speech therapist suggested starting with a broad question and then narrow it down. Thinking of broader categories, I asked, "Was it a neighbor? Was it someone from church? Did someone from the office come by?"

David shook his head each time. No, no, no as his brows furrowed.

"David, I must write a thank you note. Let's take this slow."

He put his hand up, gesturing me to stop talking. "I," he began again.

"I?" I repeated. "I can't think of anyone whose name starts with the letter 'I'," I said, feeling defeated.

Finally, as words failed him, David thought of another way to communicate. While he was as frustrated as I was, he had an idea. He opened the dishwasher. Inside, there were the tell tale signs that the cookies were made in my own kitchen. I smiled as I looked down at my son, the mystery baker.

David, with his face beaming, repeated simply. "I," he repeated.

'I, indeed!" I said with a joy I hadn't felt in weeks.

David proved that he could do things by himself and he did not need my constant help. He wanted to surprise us and had even painstakingly lined the basket with a cloth napkin--and managed it all one-handedly.

I learned a valuable lesson that night. Had David asked me (by pantomime and gestures) if he could bake cookies while we were away, I would have said a very firm, *No.* Yet, there were many things David was capable of doing and it was important to focus on what he *could* do, not on what he couldn't.

◇ ◇ ◇

> *"Focus on what you can do. Not on what you cannot do."* David Dow

Hope

There is much to be hopeful for. Aphasia caused by a stroke or brain injury is not a terminal or progressive disease that gets worse over time. People continue to make progress for years after their diagnosis. Just because your speech therapy benefits have ended for the year doesn't mean your recovery limitations should. There are many resources available to you through support groups, Facebook, computer software, therapy apps, workbooks, to use at home and university clinics. In fact, sometimes there are so many options that it is overwhelming. Take your time. Educate yourself. Learn what your insurance covers and day by day you will get through this. And find the best fits for you and your family.

You may have been told that aphasia improvement only occurs in the first 6 months or year after your stroke or brain injury. Some therapists use the term *plateau* to describe when they feel you may have reached your maximum recovery potential. However, there is increasing evidence that recovery continues to occur years and even decades after the initial diagnosis of aphasia.[lxiii] It is actually normal that there are times you will not see the process. What we don't want to happen is times when you stop working or caring. It's hard to continue when you do not see progress, but finding ways to communicate and using strategies will help you manage the rest of your life with tools rather than just giving up!

There is a growing consensus among Speech-Language Pathologists that a plateau in aphasia recovery does not exist. Typically, the "spontaneous recovery period" can last up to two years where someone with aphasia will often make the most progress.[lxiv] But, people with aphasia can and do continue to make progress. Many report some gains ten or more years after their initial diagnosis if they have continued to challenge themselves to promote neuroplasticity.

David is a good example of continued progress. He did not expect to see significant gains in year six. However, he participated in an intensive program where he received daily speech therapy, sometimes twice a day. He made amazing gains because he was challenging himself throughout the day. While his case may seem unusual, many ARC members have similar experiences. When challenged with intensive work, they find they can and do make gains. Many insurance companies do not cover services for high intensity therapy programs, however, some families do fundraising to help cover these costs.

You and your family need to make choices best for you, your budget, and your lifestyle. Remember, there are many low cost ways you can challenge yourself. But it takes a lot of discipline, support, and help from others along the way.

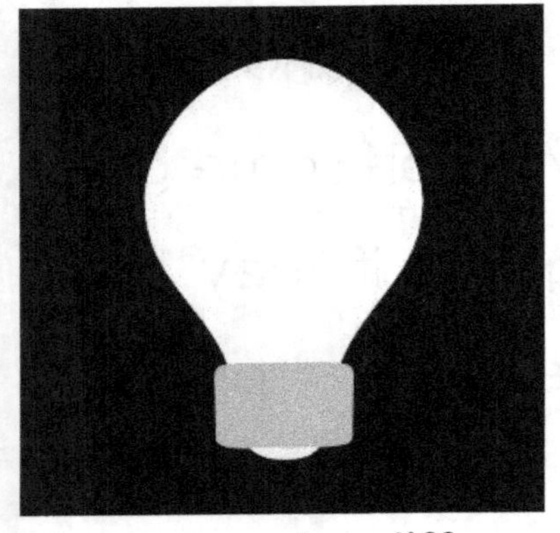

Aphasia Tip

If somebody tells you that you have reached a plateau in therapy, ask what you can do differently in therapy to challenge yourself.

Also, ask yourself if you are dedicated and determined right now. Sometimes, you may just need a break. And that is OK. This is a huge adjustment. Don't feel guilty. You are human. You can take a break. Re-group. And plan to go back to therapy later.

Perhaps the exercises you were doing in therapy lacked variety and you need more real life situations to make further improvement.

Ask to focus on different goals or use different techniques such as Melodic Intonation Therapy or incorporate technology into treatment.

Therapy should also include real life goals that are of interest to you. Such as: planning a trip, calling a loved one, reading a favorite book or recipe.

We have found that there are times therapists use the term plateau because therapy benefits have ended although your potential for recovery has not. Perhaps your therapist does not specialize in aphasia therapy and you could benefit from a therapist with more experience with aphasia therapy. That is not to say you don't have a good therapist. But, we believe that therapists that continue to push you and believe in you are best for your recovery. The positive energy and coaching that comes from your therapist is often key to your motivation.

Many therapists also specialize in various fields of speech therapy. ARC members often share that they prefer to have a therapist who specializes in aphasia therapy. Carol often uses the term, there are some therapists that are often

#AphasiaJunkies. They are the ones often focusing specifically on aphasia with continued learning and dedication to this particular focus. Other therapists have other special interests. It is not a reflection on your therapist. Just like teachers – some specialize.

You have the ability to continue to make progress on your own. Speech therapy isn't magic and language recovery can happen throughout your day with continued effort on your part to challenge yourself.

> **Speech-Language Pathologist Dr. Lori Bartels-Tobin of The Aphasia Center in St. Petersburg, FL. explains, "Do not let anyone claim that stroke survivors cannot get better. Become empowered. Be insistent. It might take more time and effort, but it can be done. Get started now."[1] Her center focuses only on aphasia treatment.**

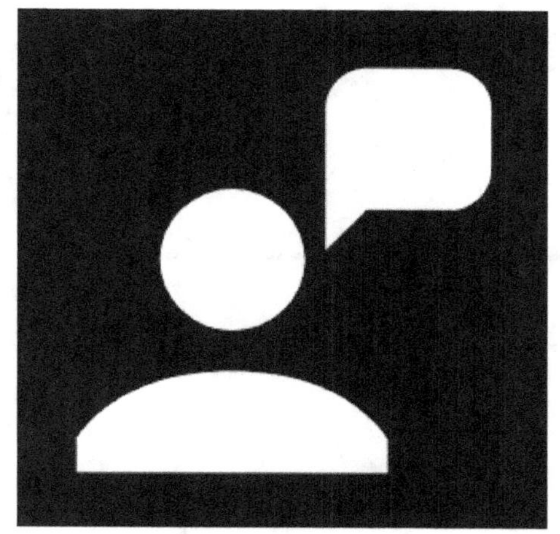

Self Evaluation

➢ **What gives me hope?**

____

____

____

____

____

➢ **How can I tell someone how I am feeling?**

____

____

____

____

➢ **What can I do if someone says I have reached a plateau in my recovery?**

____

____

➢ **Do I need a break?**

____

____

➢ **Do I feel my speech therapist believes in me? Is my SLP an aphasia specialist?**

____

____

➢ **Do I want help for my emotions? Do I want to talk to a doctor about it?**

____

____

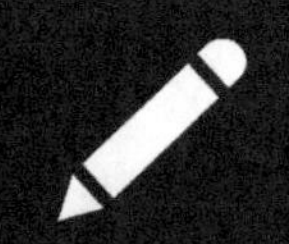

> **What Are Some Other Ways Of Communicating Without Talking?**

People with aphasia can learn how to improve communication using aphasia communication compensatory strategies. Make sure to try every mode of communication. If it works for you, then it's an excellent strategy! Writing, gestures, pointing, singing, reading, using picture cards, or communication technology are all viable options to improve communication.

Carol shares this account: A few years ago, I was on a tour off a cruise ship right after departure. I noticed a man who appeared to be a stroke survivor. He had right-sided paralysis like my son David. I approached him, introduced myself, and asked him for his name. Silence. (As I thought might happen.)

I proceeded to ask him if he could spell his name.

Yes, he nodded.

I opened the palm of my hand for him to draw the letter. Using his finger, he drew the letter J. "John? Jim? Jack?" I asked.

YES! He nodded. His name was Jack.

Later, I saw Jack seated at dinner with his wife. I went to his table, introduced myself, and said, "Hi Jack. This must be your wife."

She glared at me. "How do you know my husband's name?" she demanded. "He can't talk!" She seemed very angry.

"I met Jack on the tour this morning," I told her.

"But he CANNOT TALK!" she insisted.

"Perhaps not," I said. "But he CAN communicate."

Often, we think of aphasia recovery only about regaining speech. However success in recovery also means finding new ways to communicate. It means adapting. And finding recovery also means finding new ways to find success in communicating—like my friend Jack. We spent much of our cruise together while David and Jack bonded and we supported Jack's communication.

Later, the wife confided in me that she'd pretty much, "given up." But, she was able to engage in several days with our family as we helped support Jack and she learned that Jack was, indeed, very capable. But it was going to take more effort on her part to learn the appropriate strategies for her husband to find success. (Success sometimes means adapting to change).

Sometimes seemingly both Speech-Language Pathologist and caregivers can miss obvious modes of communication. If there is something you can do that your family doesn't know about, try your best to let them know.

An ARC member shared her experience that emphasizes the importance of trying every mode of communication early on. She shares:

"I didn't know for a year that my husband could read. One day my husband got agitated while I was on the computer. He hit the caps key and started banging the keyboard. It suddenly dawned on me that he wanted either to type or have me write in uppercase. I can't tell you what a new world it opened up to us. My husband now reads about ten pages a day. He is starting to understand lowercase and if he doesn't, I write it in uppercase for him."

Another ARC member shared this advice for people who have just been diagnosed with aphasia:

"Be kind to yourself, you've been through a trauma. You might be tired, you might find that your emotions are out of control. But, you will want to use any means you can to communicate. Paper, pen, photos, gestures, whatever works for you. Rest if you can. Give yourself time."

Strategies for People with Aphasia

When meeting new people, it will be helpful to let them know you have aphasia. There are cards that you can purchase that explain that aphasia impacts language but not intelligence. You can make your own card and personalize it with things that help improve communication. Here is an example:

> **I Have Aphasia (From a Stroke):**
>
> This means I have difficulty with communication.
>
> Please give me time to express myself.
>
> I can write down what I want to say.
>
> Aphasia doesn't impact my intelligence.

The Aphasia Center's website has free pocket aphasia cards that you can customize and print out. Find them here: **theaphasiacenter.com/pocket-card**

Getting stuck on a particular word is one of the most common symptoms of aphasia. The key is to try your best not to get frustrated. Take a deep breath and think of other ways to say what you want. Don't get too focused on the word. There are other ways to get your point across.

This moment is a perfect opportunity to build new neural pathways by using other modes of communication.

Describing the word, gesturing, making sound effects, saying colors, location or writing the word are all options to communicate what you want to say.

Aphasia Tip

When you get stuck on a particular word, it is useful to think of descriptive cues to communicate your point. Try to answer these questions:

➢ Where do you find it?

➢ What do you use it for?

➢ When do you use it?

➢ Who uses it?

➢ Why do you use it?

➢ How could you use it?

➢ Show a gesture of yourself using it.

➢ Can you share the first letter of the word?

➢ What sound does it make?

When somebody with aphasia is stuck on a particular word, it is hard to take a deep breath and step back from focusing solely on the word itself and think of other ways you can express what you are trying to say. Most people with aphasia will tell you, the more anxious you get, the harder it becomes. So – take that deep breath.

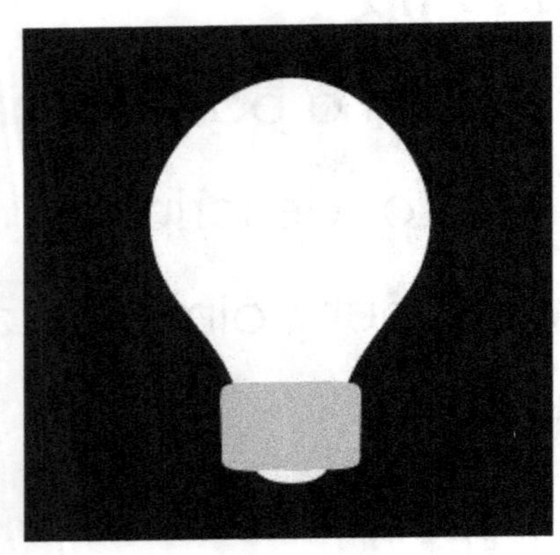

Aphasia Tip

Some great ways to express yourself:

o Singing

o Drawing

o Writing

o Pointing

o Facial Expressions

o Gestures

Use whatever works!

One ARC member offers this advice: "Use as many senses as you can. Read out loud. Sing to the tune *Happy Birthday* as you read the words. Bake cookies. Read the newspaper out loud. Have someone read the newspaper to you and discuss it. Look at family pictures and tell family stories. Put closed captioning on TV. Make letters out of sandpaper and trace the words you make with the letters as you say them."

Virtual Connections (the Zoom program by Lingraphica and ARC) offers sessions by music therapists. Often, the therapist sings, "Where are you from?" then, the attendee is often able to sing the answer back, while they may struggle to say the city, when put to music, they often can sing, "I'm from _______," when modeled by the music therapist.

ARC members understand that communication can be exhausting. Determination to express yourself is key. Even if what you want to say is a small thing, every time you push yourself to communicate it is one step further in your rehabilitation. We encourage you to join ARC so you can chat with others going through this journey. You are not alone.

We also encourage care partners to be cautious of being critical. This is hard work. It takes small steps. It's best to be an encourager and not over-correct and criticize. All too often, if criticized too often, that is the first step for a person with aphasia to stop trying.

It may take takes longer to express yourself. Both you and those you love are going to be practicing patience on this road to recovery. Most people with aphasia experience well-meaning people who will attempt to finish your sentence for you. If this happens, try to say the word anyway and then say something like, "Thanks, but I can do it." Or, put your hand up signaling the other person to stop and wait. The more you try, the better.

Carol shares lightheartedly that aphasia sometimes looks like a head-turned disease. That is because all too often the person with aphasia turns their head, looking for someone to do the talking. While this may be necessary for some in the beginning, it is important that you break this habit and try as much as you are capable of to get the words out.

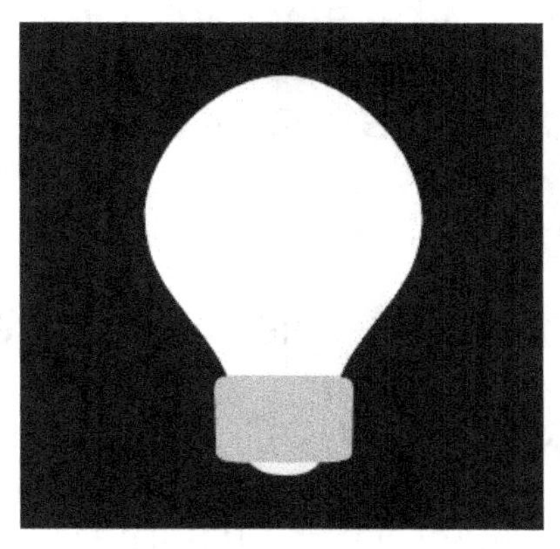

Aphasia Tip

➤ Practice saying a phrase that will help you during conversations such as: "Just give me a minute."

➤ "Give me a second, I can say it."

➤ "I know it. I just need to find the word."

➤ You could put your hand up firmly, gesturing for them to stop.

➤ You need to take ownership and you will indeed have times where you want the other person to just stop guessing and simply give you time to try to get the word out.

➤ To improve your comprehension, don't hesitate to ask somebody to repeat what they said.

> If writing down key points helps you, carry a white board with you that says at the top, "please write that down".

> If you are able to understand what you read better than what you hear, you can use a whiteboard or a notepad app on a smartphone or tablet to have somebody write down what they said.

Adjusting to using your communication strategies will take time. It is important that you learn to use them and not shy away from asking for accommodations because of pride or embarrassment. True friends will understand and be there for you, but first, you need to give them the chance.

Communication Environment

The setting where you're trying to communicate can make a big difference on your ability to understand and express yourself. Try to limit distractions and background noise. Turn off the television and any background music. Make sure you can see the other person's face, which will help with comprehension. Try to reduce background noise because even small visual and auditory distractions can negatively impact communication. While in the hospital, remember that side conversations can be quite distracting as well.

When you are speaking to somebody with aphasia, make sure you have their full attention before you start talking. When talking to people with aphasia, do not add unnecessary details. Emphasize key words. No two people with aphasia are exactly alike, but this is generally helpful for most of us. - David Dow

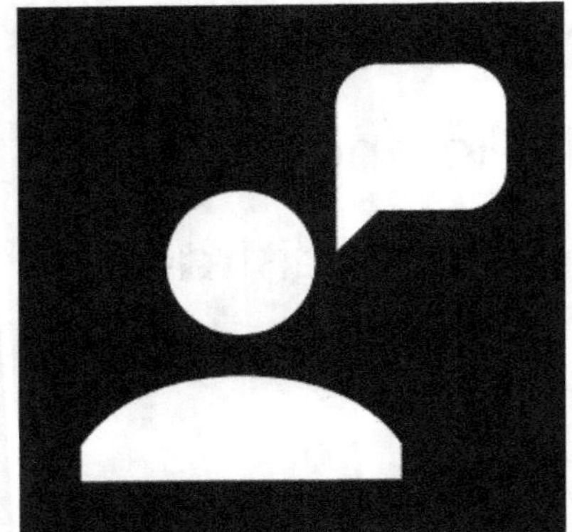

Self Evaluation

➢ **What do I wish my caregiver knew?**

____

____

____

____

➢ **What communication approaches work best for me?**

____

____

➢ **Does background noise bother me?**

____

____

➢ **Do I keep tools handy such as a whiteboard?**

____

____

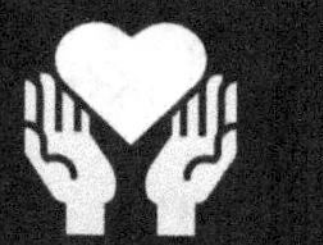

- ➢ **A Note For Caregivers**
- ➢ **Communication Tips For Caregivers**
- ➢ **Support Tips For Caregivers**
- ➢ **ARC For Caregivers**

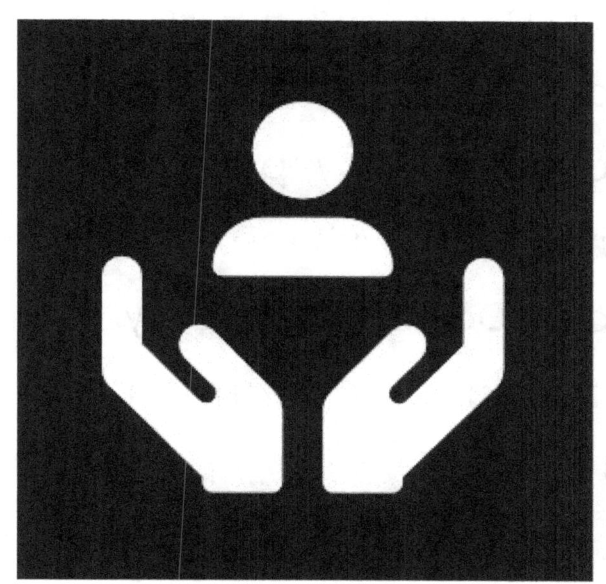

It is essential that loved ones and good friends learn tips for aphasia. Communication is a two-way street.

Carol recalls David being so frustrated for years, as she was. "I think we both cried every day for years. Aphasia is tough on you and your loved ones." While this section is devoted to your loved ones to teach them how to best help you, Carol shares a story of her early days of being a caregiver.

"Like many new caregivers, I was fumbling for solutions. Often, the TV was on—as I didn't realize that the background noise was making it so difficult for David while he was in the hospital. I would hover over David and constantly ask him yes-or-no questions. *Squeeze my hand for yes,* I'd say. *Do you want a blanket? Are you thirsty?* In fact, I developed a list of possibilities and would read it so I would not forget any possible issues he may want to communicate with me.

"One particular afternoon, David was really frustrated. I'd read the entire list and he never squeezed my hand. Finally, I said, *oh you want me to just be quiet?* David squeezed my hand so hard it hurt. So, with that, I give you the number one rule many people with aphasia want you to know: Sometimes they just want peace and quiet. They hate background noise."

Helpful tips for Caregivers

- o Speak slow and steady
- o Set a topic in the beginning
- o Stay on one topic at a time
- o Keep is simple. Eliminate unnecessary information
- o Offer choices rather than open ended questions
- o Repeat or emphasize key words
- o Write down important information or key words
- o Use simple gestures
- o Try not to talk too much with your hands.
- o Do not pretend to understand if you do not.
- o Recap the conversation for understanding.
- o Start with a broad topic then narrow it down.
- o Patience, Patience, Patience
- o Ask them if they want you to guess.
- o Do not finish the person's sentences. Provide clues or ask them to gesture or write if they can.
- o Remove background noise (TV, music, other people talking)

If you would like to learn more tips and examples, check out ARC's Top Ten Tips for Caregivers, Family, and Friends on our Aphasia Recovery Connection You Tube Channel.

To improve comprehension for someone with aphasia, speak at a slow and steady pace. You do not need to speak louder unless they are hard of hearing. Before starting a conversation, set the topic and let them know what you are going to talk about. Repeat key points. Write down important points using a whiteboard or notepad. Use simple and clear gestures when you talk to help clarify your point. Try not to talk too much with your hands because it can be distracting.

Get in the habit of keeping a notepad or whiteboard with you so you can write or draw as needed. Notepads are helpful to write and draw for both you and the person with aphasia. As mentioned earlier, many with aphasia like the inexpensive Boogie Board writing board, which is very inexpensive.

Try to keep your subject to one topic at a time. Pause slightly between sentences and let them know if the topic is going to change. You can also give them a verbal or hand gesture clue to help change topics.

Don't pretend to understand when you really don't know what the person with aphasia is trying to say. It isn't helpful to you or your loved one to pretend what they said made sense. Recap after they speak to make sure you understand correctly.

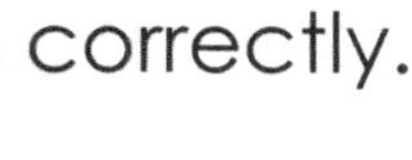

If a person with aphasia is having difficulty finding the right word, do not finish their sentence for them. Instead, provide cues to help them communicate their point. Ask if there is a gesture they can use to explain what they mean. If they can write, ask them to write or draw what they mean. Frustration is a natural aspect of anomia and expressive aphasia. If the person with aphasia gets frustrated, you can always come back to that thought in a few minutes and move on with the conversation.

If you find yourself guessing what someone with aphasia is trying to say, first try to make sure you are both talking about the same thing. Start with a broad category and then slowly narrow the subject down as you get information.

Patience for both of you is important. If conversations get exhausting, try an activity that you can enjoy without having to talk. Some board games or card games require little language and would offer a nice break. Just because somebody has aphasia doesn't mean they want to be left alone.

It is important to know whether the person wants your help or not. If you think you know what they want to say, you might ask, "Would you like me to guess?" Give the person with aphasia the chance to ask for or deny assistance. All too often family members jump in, while the person with aphasia really wants to try to get it out. And it is crucial for their recovery to allow them to try—if they want to.

Carol shares a story she learned from Natasha, a person with aphasia. She and her mom often struggled and frustration ensued. Finally, they came up with an agreed solution. They started with a scale of 1-10, asking how important is this? If it was critical, and Natasha said it was a value of 10 in important, her mom knew that in the beginning.

As a caregiver herself, Carol reminds caregivers, "Don't over help. While you may think you are helping when you jump in and take over, the reality is that the person with aphasia should try if they can and if they want to. Encourage the person with aphasia to use strategies.

As care partners, we need to empower the person with aphasia to ask when they want our help – and not just jump in and finish their sentences. I have seen many caregivers at our events that just jump right in and do all the talking. I remind them to count to 10 before they jump in. And let the person with aphasia ask for help if they want it. They have lost enough – and we need to lovingly support and encourage them, without overcorrecting and discouraging them."

Language Stimulation

Carol recalls the neurologist coming in and out of David's hospital room, saying very little. One day she ran after the doctor. Just as he was about to enter the elevator, she yelled, "Stop!" He looked stunned.

"If this was your family member, what would you do?" she asked.

"Stimulate. Stimulate and challenge David to fight for his recovery. He has to try things, even if they are hard. That is the way to recovery."

Caregivers may be able to help improve language function at home. You do not have to be a speech therapist to help your loved one with aphasia with their recovery. The life participation approach to aphasia supports the idea that family members can help optimize recovery during everyday communication and activities. Family members can play a huge role in recovery. ARC offers an additional Facebook group for caregivers to provide feedback on ways you can help with language rehabilitation at home.

Speech therapy can focus on the interests of people with aphasia. If your family member with aphasia loves sports, animals or movies, make that the focus of conversation. Try to fill your activities with language throughout the day.

You should not dwell on the mistakes, but instead focus on the positives. Do not criticize errors. After the person with aphasia says one or two words such as, "want up" model the correct sentence form and say "Okay, great. You want to get up."

Family members have the advantage of providing stimulation for language therapy in short intervals. Every time you speak together is an opportunity for improvement. Speech Therapy sessions can be long and exhausting especially for people with aphasia. Family members can stimulate speech all day long in short, manageable segments throughout the day. You can alternate between structured exercises and everyday conversation tasks.

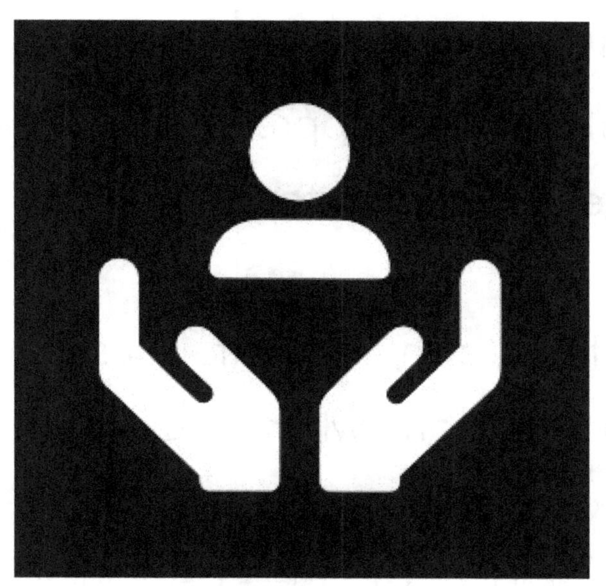

The question: "What would you like for lunch?" can be expanded into an opportunity to target descriptive language. Have them describe to you the steps involved in making a sandwich or the ingredients that you will use when you cook dinner. Have the person with aphasia read the directions from the cookbook for something that you are going to make, even if you have made it a thousand times and do not need to hear the directions. Enjoyable everyday language activities can be the best type of speech therapy.

Support

We are aware that aphasia and whatever caused the aphasia is something that happened to the entire family unit. You will hear a lot of people saying things like "take care of yourself" or "I'm here if you need me," or "What can I do to help?" But besides appreciating the platitudes, what can those friends and extended family members do?

When someone asks how they can help, it is useful to have a list and be able to tell them what you need. Some caregivers have offered advice on what they either had or wished they had, especially at the beginning of their journey.

Caregivers Friends and Family "What I need list."

- Household repairs

- Housework

- Yard or gardening work

- Laundry

- Shovel the snow

- Take the car for an oil change

- Gift cards for gas

- Someone to watch your loved one for a couple hours so you could have a nap or errand break.

- Bring a meal or pick up some groceries/pet food

- Take your loved one to non-medical appointments like getting a hair cut

- Can they spend time with your loved one? Perhaps they share a hobby or interest?

- Take your loved one out for a car ride or ice cream

- Help with your unique situation – ex: if you or your person with aphasia has a business, some help with that angle

- Organizational help: bills, mail, calendar

- Walk pets or pet care

Tips for Families with Children

- Babysitting

- Take the kids to their sports or watch them during a therapy/ speech appointment

- Take kids to appointments/school activities

- Anything from the previous list

You're Not Alone

You and your family do not have to face aphasia alone. Aphasia Recovery Connection is a vibrant community of people with aphasia, caregivers and Speech-Language Pathologist eager to support you in your journey of recovery. ARC and its members are available to answer your questions online or offer many of the resources you need.

ARC understands the unique journey that every individual with aphasia experiences and welcomes you with open arms. ARC "gets it," because they, too, have lived with the grief and anguish that aphasia has brought you and your loved ones. We have a Facebook Group for Caregivers. You are not alone on this journey. Learn more about ARC in the next Chapter.

Self Evaluation Caregiver:

> **What will help my loved one most as we travel the road of recovery?**

____

____

____

____

➤ **How can I stimulate language and communication skills?**

____

____

____

➤ **Might I benefit from joining ARC's Care Partner and Friends Facebook Group to find support for myself as a caregiver?**

____

____

____

➤ **What is on my list for family and friends to help with?**

____

____

____

____

> **What Is The Aphasia Recovery Connection (ARC)?**

> **How Can ARC Help My Family?**

> **What Are The ARC Facebook Page And Groups?**

> **What Are Some Other Things ARC Is Doing?**

> **How Can I Help ARC?**

"ARC is a lifeline for people with aphasia who struggle to communicate. It's a place to find their voice and find others on the journey."
Cheryl P, FL

What is the

Aphasia Recovery Connection (ARC)?

ARC offers lifeline for families dealing with aphasia as an award-winning nonprofit organization. ARC was founded by David and his mom Carol who you met throughout the pages of this book.

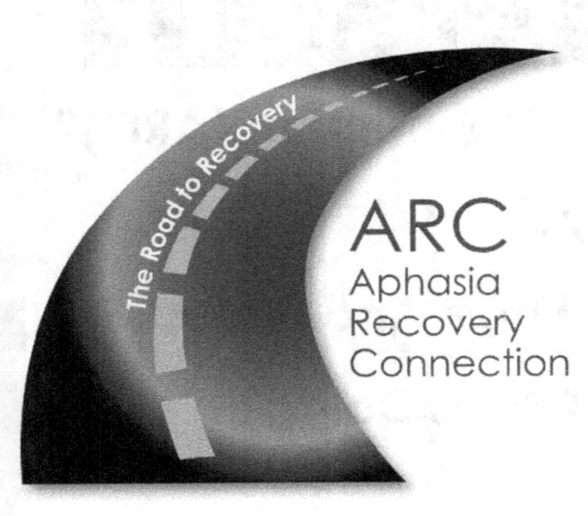

ARC brings families together with rehab professionals to learn, share, and connect online and at events.ARC received the RAISE *Award* from the National Stroke Association for making an impact on the lives of stroke survivors. They are frequent speakers at the American Speech-Language-Hearing Association (ASHA) conferences and have given presentations at Medical CME Conferences and television programs. Both Carol and David have received numerous Aphasia Advocate awards for their passion supporting families like yours.

"ARC has been a lifeline for us. Connecting with others has given us insight and hope. I've learned so much from others and the experts that post here." – a caregiver

Aphasia Recovery Connection Mission

Our mission is to deliver compassionate support services to improve the quality of life for people recovering from aphasia and their families and friends.

We are committed to helping to end the isolation that aphasia brings.

We embody the values of collaboration, compassion, dignity, and acceptance.

"The mission of ARC has allowed individuals who felt isolated and alone to find others with aphasia, and caregivers access to ideas, problem-solving and, most importantly, hope." Maura S, NC

How Can ARC Help My Family?

We believe that connecting with others can be helpful while you are navigating your aphasia journey. ARC offers support and education on Facebook, YouTube, and at events. ARC offers caregiver support groups, daily video sessions, games, and helps bring current research to you. ARC actively creates awareness with hundreds of aphasia awareness posters that are shareable and copyright free. ARC's Director, Carol Dow-Richards, often offers face-to-face sessions with Facebook Messenger Rooms.

Additionally, ARC has hosted events such as aphasia retreats, multi-day conferences, aphasia boot camps, and aphasia cruises.

"ARC is providing a service that does not exist anywhere else. People all over the US and beyond its borders are benefiting. The information the organization provides to people with aphasia and their care partners is phenomenal. There is always someone to answer any questions." Barb N. NY

Join the ARC Aphasia Family

ARC's success is often summed up by its members who say, "ARC gets it." ARC "gets it" because they live it. The team believes there are three main experts on aphasia: the therapists/medical personnel, the person with aphasia, and the families. ARC successfully brings the synergy and cooperation of the groups together, which serves to help families who are often struggling with the same issues we have.

"The isolation that aphasia often brings can be alleviated by being in contact with others going through the same difficulties. The enthusiasm that ARC brings to all is wonderful. It has provided our son with a safe place to get back into public speaking. " Ann B, NC

Facebook Page and Groups

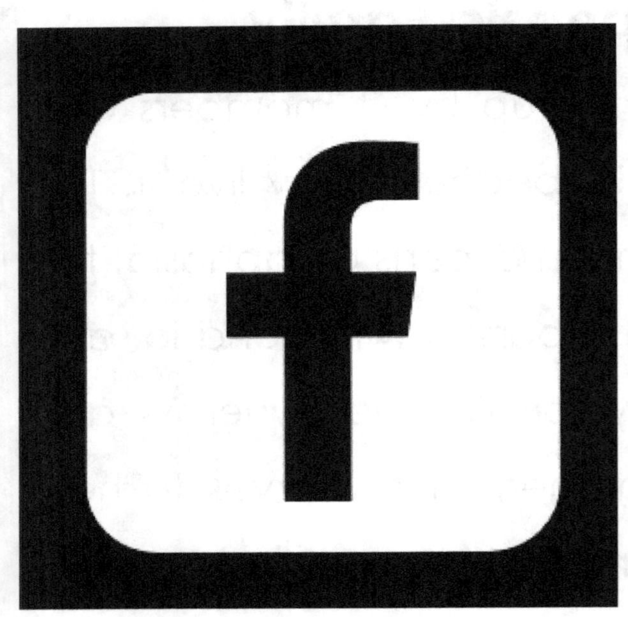

ARC started as a Facebook Book in 2012 when David, then 28, had moved to a new city and was struggling to meet others. He suggested a Facebook Group and ARC quickly became the largest and most engaged aphasia community online.

In fact, even Facebook Headquarters took notice! ARC was invited to Facebook Headquarters in 2019 to celebrate the success and learn more about Facebook's partnership to connect people throughout the world. ARC now offers a public page, a private group, a private caregiver's group, and even a kid's group.

ARC offers free online support for families right on Facebook with over 10,000 members. Their members share ideas and strategies and ask questions. There are many Speech and Language Pathologists here with us as well.

Facebook: ARC *Public Page*

The public site is for those interested in aphasia. It offers many videos as well as educational posters for people with aphasia and their friends and family members to share on their own timelines to help raise awareness with copyright free posters. You can find the public page here:

facebook.com/aphasiaARC

Facebook: ARC Facebook *Group*:

"When my daughter discovered ARC, a whole new life opened up for her. The group provides tools and resources unknown to us. They ended the isolation of aphasia

as she met more people life herself. She has been treated with dignity and recognized for her abilities. This organization helped the family to be her champion; how-to carry-on family conversations to enable her full participation." Joan S, VA

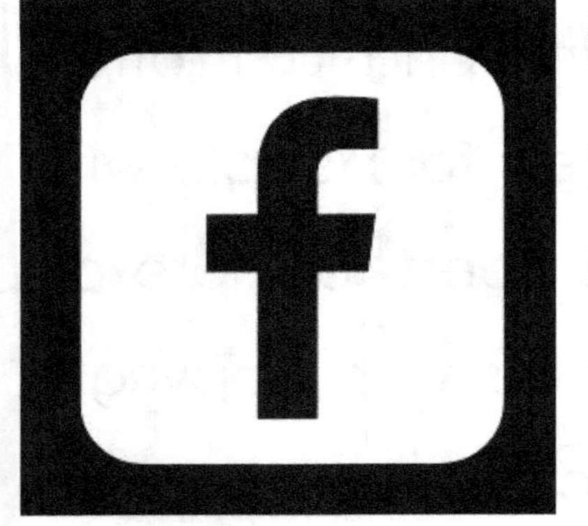

The private group site is for people with aphasia, their loved ones, and related professionals. It is not open to the general public and only members can see posts. You can request membership by going to this web address:

facebook.com/groups/Aphasia.Recovery.Connection

A detailed guide to join the Facebook group is in **Appendix D**.

Facebook: ARC Caregiver Group

This private group is for Care Partners only. It is not open to the public and only members can view posts. You can request to join at: Facebook Caregiver Group at this web address:

facebook.com/groups/ARC.Care.Partners/

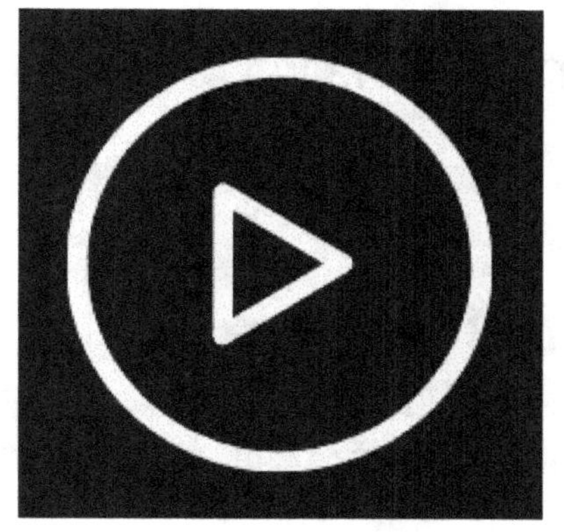

Instagram

Twitter

ARC Youtube Channel

ARC knows people with aphasia benefit from many ways to receive information and created aphasia friendly videos on a variety of topics related to aphasia. ARC Youtube Channel here: www.youtube.com/c/AphasiaRecovery Connection.

ARC on Other Social Media

Find us on **Instagram** as Aphasia Recovery Connection

Follow us on **Twitter**: @ARCaphasia

ARC Events

ARC Aphasia Cruises, Boot Camps, and events offer are offer sessions by aphasia experts. Check the website for the latest updates. www.aphasiarecoveryconnection.org

Health Care Support And Education

We offer a free webinar thru ASHA to help support those in the hospital and hospital staff.

youtu.be/_sTl5wknOug

ARC Speakers Bureau

Looking for a guest speaker at your next conference or webinar? Email us: arcteam@aphasiarecoveryconnecti on.org with your conference date, size, and location.

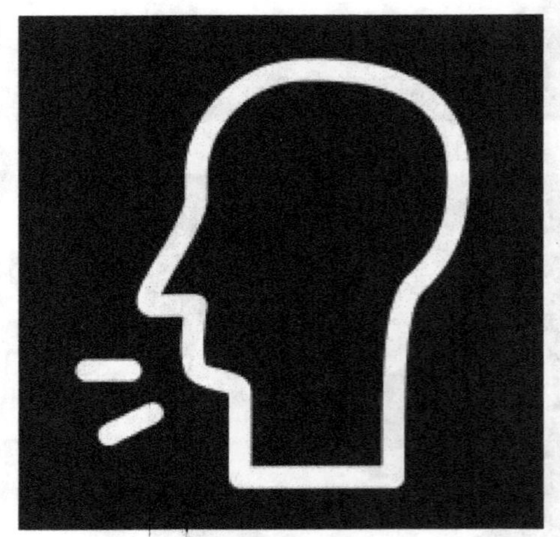

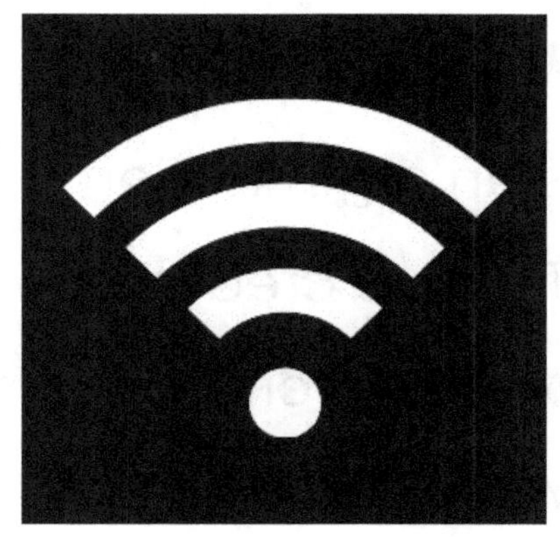

Virtual Connections Collaboration

Virtual Connections - This free video conferencing program on ZOOM is provided by ARC in collaboration with Lingraphica. *Virtual Connections* helps people with aphasia meet online with others who have aphasia and provides a safe place for all to practice their communications skills in real-time conversations. Caregiver sessions are also offered. Sessions are facilitated by speech-language pathologists, music therapists, and aphasia experts.

And, over the 2020 pandemic, they have expanded their online services to reach people in all 50 states and over 20 countries with a volunteer force of over 40 rehab professionals.

Register for an upcoming session based on your own interests. And, there is usually a caregiver session offered each week:

devices.aphasia.com/virtual-connections

CATS and ARC Collaboration

Collaboration of Aphasia Trialist, CATS is an organization of international researchers. ARC and CATS have created a Facebook research dissemination team. We are working together to create short aphasia friendly videos that will summarize key aphasia research and what their findings mean for people with aphasia. Watch and subscribe to the CATS/ARC Youtube channel here:

youtube.com/channel/UCeQhdK9vye7EPVTpIbqlSag

Aphasia Games For Health Collaboration

Aphasia Games for Health is a partnership of ARC, the University of Pittsburgh, Carnegie Mellon University, and Thorny Games. To learn more visit:

aphasiagamesforhealth.com/

Website – Join Our Mailing List

AphasiaRecoveryConnection.org

New Plans Underway

Currently, ARC is working to create downloadable and print materials for families new to aphasia. We are committed to finding ways to support families online and off, so the public is more aware and families have self-advocacy and educational materials for their communities. ARC is also involved with Project Bridge, Western Division. This project is funded by PCORI. (Patient Centered Outcomes Research Initiative) Stay tuned to ARC events on their website or on their Facebook site.

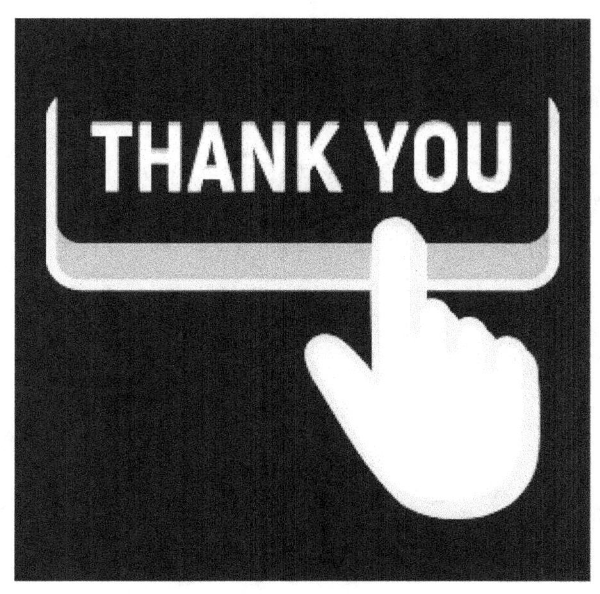

How You Can Help

As a nonprofit organization, our mission is supported by donors who are committed to aphasia awareness, aphasia advocacy, and family support.

While we reach out to

those we serve with support and education, we also ask that those we serve support the mission and help us grow if they are able.

Become A Donor: Support The Mission

www.aphasiarecoveryconnection.org/donate

Become An Aphasia
Advocate & Fundraiser

Share Your Story – Want to share your own aphasia story on Facebook while supporting ARC? Create a Facebook Fundraiser!

Go to: www.facebook.com/fund/aphasiaARC/

All Facebook Fundraisers are recognized each month on the Aphasia Recovery Connection Group Site as Aphasia Ambassadors.

Corporate Giving

Many corporations offer donor matching.

You will need our address and EIN Number:

EIN 46-4170028

10624 S. Eastern Ave., A379

Henderson, NV 89052

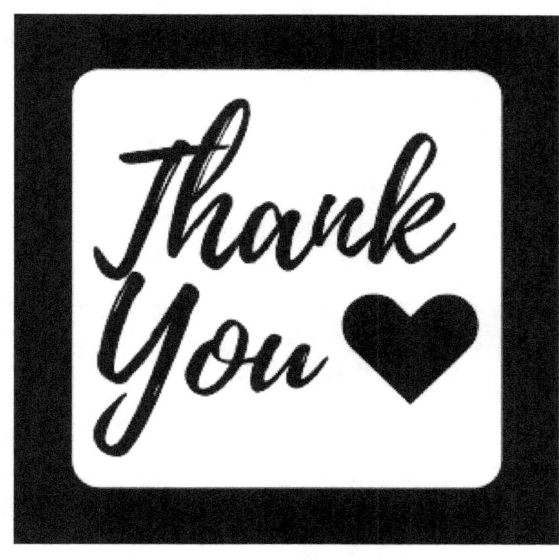

And **Thank YOU!** You already helped ARC by buying this book. Profits from the sale of this book will go to support the mission of the Aphasia Recovery Connection.

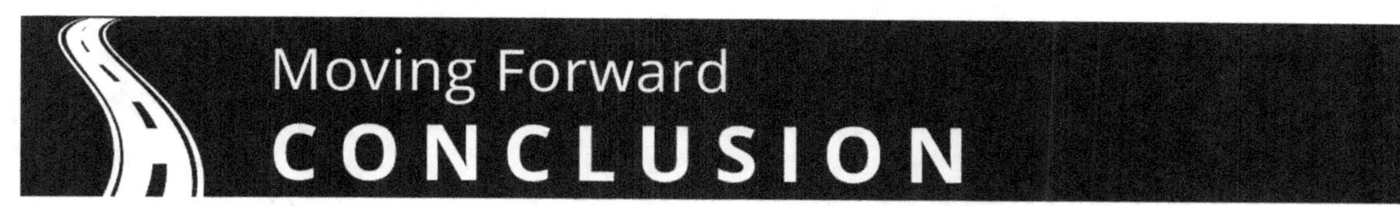

By now, you've learned a lot about aphasia and may be feeling a little overwhelmed. Take it a day at a time.

I so wish I had a magic wand. Or a magic pill. Unfortunately, recovery from aphasia takes a long time and many are left with some form of chronic aphasia for the rest of the their lives. Remember, don't compare yourself to others. What we want for you is for you to be the BEST that you can be. Your goal is to optimize your own recovery.

Often, people think of their goal like this, "I want to talk. I want to drive. I want to read." All natural desires and I'm glad you want those things.

Remember to start with small attainable goals.

If I need to lose 100 lbs., it doesn't happen overnight. It happens with small attainable goals with daily effort. What can you do today to work on a goal? It may be starting with single words. Two or three words. Spelling your name.

Take your time.

Another goal to remember is this: Recovery has 2 roads that are equally important: The road to recovery that is indeed about talking more. Reading, writing. Those are often good long-term goals. This road can be slow at first.

For David, in the beginning, it was learning to use a whiteboard and drawing to communicate. It didn't come naturally and we had to work on it - and get better. Later, it was using text-to-speech to support his reading. Even pacing yourself or practicing phrases ahead are strategies for success.

Life is short and we want you to have the best quality of life - and communication with others. This means being with others, either in person if possible or virtually if it is not possible. Finding a support system is a learning strategy too. This is also important. Using your strategies are also part of your recovery. This road to recovery is sometimes missed.

We look forward to seeing you on our Facebook Group or on a Virtual Connections chat!

We often say: If you have had a bad day - you may need us. And if you have had a good day - we need you.

ARC is a community. An aphasia family. This is one "club" you'd never ask to "join" - but here we are. Families dealing with aphasia.

You don't have to walk this journey alone.

Warmly,

Carol and David

Communication Template to use in Hospital

Have your caregiver or family help you to complete the thoughts. This will help you communicate with the people around you.

- I have aphasia.
- I worked as a: _______________
- Aphasia does not affect my intellect.
- Please talk slowly.
- Emphasize key words.
- I can read. Write down key words.
- I communicate with _____________________
- My family members are: _________________
- My hearing is fine. There is no need to yell.
- I am originally from: ________________.
- I _______________ write.
- I love to_________________ .

APPENDIX B

Helpful Links

Amanda P. Anderson M.S. CCC-SLP Aphasia Teletherapy Website: www.aphasiateletherapy.com

American Stroke Association: www.stroke.org/

AHA Stroke Prevention: www.heart.org/en/healthy-living/healthy-lifestyle/my-life-check--lifes-simple-7

Amy's Speech and Language Therapy, AAC Resources: www.amyspeechlanguagetherapy.com/communication-boards

Aphasia Access: www.aphasiaaccess.org/

Aphasia Games For Health: www.aphasiagamesforhealth.com/

Aphasia Recovery Connection Facebook page: www.facebook.com/aphasiaARC/

Aphasia Recovery Connection Website: www.aphasiarecoveryconnection.org/

Virtual Connections: https://devices.aphasia.com/virtual-connections

Aphasia Software Finder:
www.aphasiasoftwarefinder.org/

ASHA Aphasia Info:
www.asha.org/practice-portal/clinical-topics/aphasia/

ASHA Webinar:
www.youtube.com/watch?v=_sTl5wknOug

Collaboration of Aphasia Trial Lists:
www.aphasiatrials.org/

National Aphasia Association: www.aphasia.org/

Tactus Therapy: List of Aphasia Apps:
tactustherapy.com/free-list-best-speech-therapy-apps-adults/

The Aphasia Center (pocket card):
theaphasiacenter.com/pocket-card/

U.S. News World Report, Top Rehab Hospitals:
www.sci-info-pages.com/top-rehabilitation-hospitals/

Alder Aphasia Center
Maywood New Jersey
201- 368- 8585

Aphasia Center of California
Oakland California
510 -336- 0112

Aphasia Center of Tucson
Tucson, Arizona
520- 730- 8428

Aphasia Center of West Texas
Midland, Texas
432 - 699- 1261
www.aphasiawtx.org/

Aphasia Communication Enhancement Program
Kalamazoo, Michigan
269 - 387- 7000
www.wmich.edu/unifiedclinics/vanriper/aphasia/

Aphasia Institute
Toronto, Ontario, Canada
416-226-3636 ext 24
www.aphasia.ca/

Aphasia Resource Center
Boston University
617-353-0197
www.bu.edu/aphasiacenter/

Communication Recovery Groups at St. Jude
Fullerton, California
714-992-3000 ext 31

Communication Recovery Groups at CSU
Sacramento, California
916-278-6695

Dalhousie Aphasia Clinic
Halifax, Nova Scotia
902-494-5158
www.aphasiaaction.com/

Houston Aphasia Recovery Center
Houston, TX
713-781-7100
www.harctx.org/

Moss Rehab Aphasia Center
Philadelphia, PA
215-663-6554
www.mrri.org/index.php/focus-areas/

Shirley Ryan AbilityLab,
Illinois
844-355-ABLE
www.sralab.org

Snyder Center for Aphasia Life Enhancement
Baltimore, MD
410-323-1777
www.scalebaltimore.org/

Stroke Comeback Center
Vienna, Virginia
703-255-5221
www.strokecomebackcenter.org/

The Aphasia House
University of Central Florida, Orlando
407-882-0468
www.ucf.edu/

Triangle Aphasia Project Unlimited (TAPS)
Raleigh, NC
919-650-3854
www.aphasiaproject.org/

More information on the LPAA model for professionals can be found at www.AphasiaAccess.org or on the public Facebook Page for Aphasia Access.

How to join Facebook:

1. Open your web browser. Type in **facebook.com**

2. Under "Sign Up", type in your name, email address or mobile number, and create a password. You will use your email address or mobile number to log in to Facebook.

3. Select your birthday, male or female, and then click the large green tab that says "sign up".

4. On the next page, you can follow the directions to "Find your friends" on Facebook or "skip this step" by clicking the option on the bottom of the box.

5. On the next two screens, you can "Fill out info" about yourself or skip the steps.

How to join Aphasia Recovery Connection's Facebook Group

Log in to Facebook. At the top of the page you will see a box that says "Find Friends". Type "Aphasia Recovery Connection" into this box. When the ARC page appears, click "Join Group" at the top of the page.

You can do the same for any of our Facebook Groups.

ARC Aphasia Recovery Connection Care Partners & Friends

Educating family and friends is helpful, so here are some things you can share with them.

What is Aphasia?

Aphasia is a communication disability that may impact speaking, understanding, reading, and writing.   (one or a combination)

Acquired aphasia is caused by damage to the part of the brain and affects language, not intellect. Aphasia is most often from a stroke or traumatic brain injury.

Aphasia is an **invisible** – but very real – disability.

Communication takes two or more people. We believe aphasia is a **family** issue, not an issue of one person. We believe aphasia is a **community** issue, as people with aphasia participate in life in commerce, public places, and social gatherings.

From *Brain Attack*: David's Quick Helpful Tips to Share with Family and Friends

Communication Tips:

My family and friends did many things to help me because of my aphasia. Here is some advice I have for you when you talk to people with aphasia.

- **Do not treat us as if we are dumb.**
- **Talk slowly.**
- **Pause between sentences.**
- **Be patient with us.**
- **Use gestures to help us understand.**
- **Do not try to talk to us with the TV or music on.**
- **Bring pictures to share with us.**
- **Have our attention before you talk to us.**
- **Write down key words if we do not understand.**
- **Do not be critical of our mistakes. We are trying.**
- **Do not rush us.**
- **Do not make fun of the way we walk or talk.**
- **Keep a clipboard and pen nearby.**

- **Help us load aphasia apps on our smart phones or tablets.**
- **Respect us. Aphasia affects our language, not our intellect!**
- **Include us in conversations. We are not invisible.**

More Tips from David

After my stroke, a lot of things changed for me. My family and friends did a lot to help me adapt to being one-handed. These are some things you can do to help someone who has had a stroke.

- **Help us conserve energy.**
- **Find ways to help us smile, laugh, and enjoy life.**
- **Be our friends. We need you.**
- **Keep your visits short.**
- **Remember, rugs may be trip hazards.**
- **Try to be one-handed for a day.**
- **Stay hopeful. Encourage us.**
- **Help find a support group. Check online.**

- Take us out. Let us do things again.

- Do not be overprotective of us.

- Advocate for us. We need your help.

- Help us eat healthy. We do not need to gain weight!

- Let us rest. Naps are good. But don't let us be couch potatoes! We need to keep our muscles strong to improve.

- Easy crafts or things we can do in our free time.

- An internet-capable tablet is helpful to download aphasia apps and games.

- One-handed products can be found online. Look for a one-handed can-opener, a knife/fork combo, a plate with high rims, and non-slip material to put under plates and bowls.

- The best gift of all is a visit or call that leaves us encouraged and with a smile on our faces.

Things you can do to reduce the risk of additional strokes are to eat healthy and exercise. There is a wealth of information available on how to reduce your risk of stroke. The American Heart association offers an interactive risk factor assessment tool on their website:

mylifecheck.heart.org

The American Stroke Association also has information on their website (stroke.org) regarding what stroke risk factors you can control, such as high blood pressure, smoking, diabetes, carotid and other artery disease, atrial fibrillation, transient ischemic attacks, high cholesterol, physical inactivity, obesity, excessive alcohol consumption, and illegal drug use, and how to curtail the risks.[lxv]

It is important that you understand risk factors you can control to reduce stroke risks. For example, according to the American Heart Association, smoking nearly doubles your risk of ischemic stroke.[lxvi]

Fortunately, the American Heart Association reports rapid decreases in mortality rates and incidence of ischemic strokes with the immediate cessation of smoking.[lxvii] The American Stroke Association reports that within 5 years of the first stroke, the chance of having a recurrent stroke increases as much as 40%.[lxviii] Second strokes have higher death rates and more severe disabilities since part of the brain has already been injured and is not as resilient to trauma.[lxix] Become your own advocate and get proactive about your health. Find out why you had your first stroke and do everything you can to reduce your risks of having another.

If you have another stroke, knowing the symptoms and acting immediately can save your life. The National Stroke Association promotes a way to help remember the signs and symptoms of stroke:

FAST:

- **F**ace: Look in the mirror and smile or have someone check to see if one side of your face is drooping.

- **A**rm: Raise both of your arms, does one droop downwards? Does one arm feel numb or tingle?

- **S**peech: Try to say a simple sentence. Are you able to get the words out? Is your speech slurred? Does your tongue feel numb?

- **T**ime: If you present with these symptoms, call 911 immediately to receive the proper care to prevent further damage to your brain.[1]

AAC: Augmentative and Alternative Communication, typically a device that is used for communication.

ADL: Activities of Daily Living, A term used in rehabilitation referring to routine activities that people tend to do everyday without needing assistance. There are six basic ADLs: eating, bathing, dressing, toileting, transferring (walking) and continence.

AFO: Ankle-foot orthosis: A brace, usually made of plastic that is worn on the lower leg and foot to support the ankle, hold the foot and ankle in the correct position and correct foot drop. Abbreviated AFO. Also known as foot drop brace.

ALF: Assisted Living Facility, residential community that provides nursing care, rehab services, and meals for residents.

Aneurysm: bulge or ballooning in a blood vessel.

Anomia: a form of aphasia in which the patient is unable to recall the names of everyday objects.

Aphasia: Aphasia is an impairment of language, affecting the production or comprehension of speech and the ability to read or write resulting from injury to the brain.

ASHA: American Speech-Language-Hearing Association (ASHA) is the national professional, scientific, and credentialing association for more than 173,070 members and affiliates who are audiologists; speech-language pathologists; speech, language, and hearing scientists; audiology and speech-language pathology support personnel; and students.

Aspiration Pneumonia: Pneumonia caused by food or liquid entering the airway and lungs as a result of dysphagia. Stroke survivors are at high risk for aspiration pneumonia, which can be life threatening.

Brain Hemorrhage: A type of stroke. It is caused by an artery in the brain bursting and causing localized bleeding in the surrounding tissues. This bleeding kills brain cells.

Brain Lesion: abnormal areas of tissue in the brain.

Carotid Artery Dissection: is a separation of the layers of the artery wall supplying oxygen-bearing blood to the head and brain, and is the most common cause of stroke in young adults.

Circumlocutions: Talking around a word. Describing and using other words to explain what you are trying to say. This is actually a very positive technique and should be encouraged as a compensatory strategy.

CT Scan: A term for CAT scan, which stands for computerized axial tomography scan. A CAT scan is a painless X-ray test where a computer takes cross-section views of your anatomy. Iodine contrast can be used to view the integrity of your artery walls and blood flow.

COTA: Certified Occupational Therapy Assistant. Requires an associate's degree.

Dysphagia: Difficulty swallowing.

Inpatient: Residential rehabilitation setting either in a hospital or skilled nursing facility.

Jargon: Fluent utterances that make little or no sense, often seen in receptive aphasia.[lxx]

Life Participation Approach to Aphasia (LPAA): a consumer-driven service-delivery approach that supports individuals with aphasia and others affected by it in achieving their immediate and longer term life goals.[lxxi]

MBS: Modified Barium Swallow. Procedure used to image the swallowing process. The patient consumes foods of varying consistencies that have been coated with barium to check for aspiration and risk of choking on a variety of liquid consistencies and food textures.

MRI: Magnetic resonance imaging is a technique that uses a magnetic field and radio waves to create detailed images of the brain to show location and size of injury.

M.S. CCC-SLP: Found after a speech therapist's name. M.S stands for Master's degree in Science, CCC stands for Certificate of Clinical Competence by the American Speech-Language-Hearing Association, and SLP stands for Speech-Language Pathologist.

Moyamoya Disease: is a rare hereditary condition in which certain arteries in the brain are constricted. Blood flow is blocked by the constriction, and also by blood clots.

NAA: National Aphasia Association (aphasia.org)

NPO: Nothing by mouth.

OT: Occupational therapy: Occupational therapists apply their specific knowledge to enable people to engage in activities of daily living that have personal meaning and value. They focus on fine motor muscles and typically treat contractures and arm and hand muscle weakness for stroke survivors. Requires a Master's degree or clinical doctorate.

Outpatient: Non-residential rehabilitation setting in which you would receive therapy on an appointment basis.

Perseveration: The repetition of a particular response, such as a word, phrase, or gesture, despite the absence or cessation of a stimulus, usually a symptom of aphasia.

Phonemic Paraphasia: Substituting, adding or rearranging the speech sounds in a word.

PET SCAN: A positron emission tomography, A PET scan uses a radioactive drug (tracer) to show how your tissues and organs are functioning.

PM&R: Physical medicine and rehabilitation, also called physiatry, is the branch of medicine emphasizing the prevention, diagnosis, and treatment of disorders that are particularly related to the nerves, muscles, and bones. These disorders that may produce temporary or permanent impairment.

PO: By mouth.

Power of Attorney: POA is a written authorization that gives someone permission to act legally on your behalf in financial, medical or legal matters.

Premorbid: before the symptoms of disease or disorder.

Pseudobulbar affect (PBA): is a condition that's characterized by episodes of sudden uncontrollable and inappropriate laughing or crying. Pseudobulbar affect typically occurs in people with certain neurological conditions or injuries, which might affect the way the brain controls emotion.

PT: Physical therapists, licensed health care professionals who can help patients reduce pain and improve or restore mobility. PTs evaluate and treat gross motor (large motor) muscle deficits and help stroke survivors with strengthening, transfers and mobility. Requires a Master's degree or clinical doctorate.

PTA: Physical therapist assistant. Requires an Associates degree.

PWA: Person with aphasia.

Semantic Paraphasia: Substituting an incorrect word for another with or without recognizing the mistake.

Skype: a software application and online service that enables voice and video phone calls over the internet.

SLP: Speech-language pathologists identify, evaluate, and treat speech and language problems, including swallowing disorders. Requires a Masters degree.

SNF: Skilled Nursing Facility, an inpatient facility that provides nursing care and rehabilitation services on either a short term or long term care basis.

TBI: Traumatic Brain Injury is damage to the brain from an external mechanical force possibly leading to temporary or permanent impairment of cognitive and/or physical function.

✔ Quoted Sources
END NOTES

i American Heart Association. (2012) Let's Talk About Stroke and Aphasia, Retrieved from http://www.strokeassociation.org/idc/groups/heart-public/@wcm/@hcm/documents/downloadable/ucm_309703.pdf

ii National Institute for Neurological Disorders and Stroke (February 14, 2014). NINDS Aphasia Information Page. Retrieved from http://www.ninds.nih.gov/disorders/aphasia/aphasia.htm.

iii The American Heart Association (2014) Types of Strokes. Retrieved from http://www.strokeassociation.org/STROKEORG/AboutStroke/TypesofStroke/Types-of-Stroke_UCM_308531_SubHomePage.jsp

iv National Institute of Neurological Disorders and Stroke (2014) Ischemic Stroke. Retrieved from http://www.strokecenter.org/patients/about-stroke/ischemic-stroke/

v American Heart Association. (2014) Hemorrhagic Strokes (Bleeds). Retrieved from http://www.strokeassociation.org/STROKEORG/AboutStroke/TypesofStroke/HemorrhagicBleeds/Hemorrhagic-Strokes-Bleeds_UCM_310940_Article.jsp

vi National Heart Lung and Blood Institute. (2014) What is a Stroke? Retrieved from http://www.nhlbi.nih.gov/health/health-topics/topics/stroke/printall-index.html

vii American Heart Association. (2014) Hemorrhagic Strokes (Bleeds). Retrieved from http://www.strokeassociation.org/STROKEORG/AboutStroke/TypesofStroke/HemorrhagicBleeds/Hemorrhagic-Strokes-Bleeds_UCM_310940_Article.jsp

[viii]National Aphasia Association (2020) Aphasia FAQS.   Retrieved from: Aphasia Fact sheet HYPERLINK "http://www.aphasia.org/content/aphasia-faq"

[ix]National Aphasia Association (2020) Aphasia FAQS. Retrieved from: Aphasia Fact sheet HYPERLINK "http://www.aphasia.org/content/aphasia-faq"

[x] National Aphasia Association (2020) Aphasia FAQS. Retrieved from: https://www.aphasia.org/aphasia-resources/aphasia-factsheet/

National Aphasia Association (2011) Aphasia FAQS. Retrieved from: HYPERLINK "http://www.aphasia.org/content/aphasia-faq" http://www.aphasia.org/content/aphasia-faq

[xii] Simmons-Mackie, N. (2018) Aphasia in North America. Retrieved from: https://www.aphasiaaccess.org/white-papers/

Helm-Estabrooks, N, Albert, Martin L. (1991). Manual of Aphasia Therapy. Austin Texas: Pro-ed.

[xiv]Helm-Estabrooks, N, Albert, Martin L. (1991). Manual of Aphasia Therapy. Austin Texas: Pro-ed.

[xv]UMN Communication Science department. Retrieved from: HYPERLINK "http://www.d.umn.edu/~mmizuko/2230/sym.htm" http://www.d.umn.edu/~mmizuko/2230/sym.htm

Lazar, M. R., Antoniello, D. (November, 2008). Variability in recovery from aphasia. Current

[xvi] Neurology and Neuroscience reports, 8(6). Retrieved from http://link.springer.com/article/10.1007/s11910-008-0079-x#page-1

[xvii] Helm-Estabrooks, N, Albert, Martin L. (1991). Manual of Aphasia Therapy. Austin Texas: Pro-ed.

[xviii] Lazar, M. R., Antoniello, D. (November, 2008). Variability in recovery from aphasia. Current

Neurology and Neuroscience reports, 8(6). Retrieved from http://link.springer.com/article/10.1007/s11910-008-0079-x#page-1

[xix]Lazar, M. R., Antoniello, D. (November, 2008). Variability in recovery from aphasia. Current

Neurology and Neuroscience reports, 8(6). Retrieved from http://link.springer.com/article/10.1007/s11910-008-0079-x#page-1

[xx]National Aphasia Association. (2011). Aphasia Facts. Retrieved from: http://www.aphasia.org/content/aphasia-faq.

[xxi]Center For Disease Control and Prevention (2014). Cerebrovascular Disease or Stroke. Retrieved from http://www.cdc.gov/nchs/fastats/stroke.htm

[xxii]National Stroke Association (2014) Rehabilitation Therapy After a Stroke. Retrieved from http://www.stroke.org/site/PageServer?pagename=REHABT

[xxiii] American Stroke Association (March, 2013) Difficulty Swallowing After Stroke Dysphagia. Retrieved from http://www.strokeassociation.org/STROKEORG/LifeAfterStroke/RegainingIndependence/CommunicationChallenges/Difficulty-Swallowing-After-Stroke-Dysphagia_UCM_310084_Article.jsp.

xxiv Arcadian, CC-BY, Source: http://commons.wikimedia.org/wiki/File:Illu01_head_neck.jpg

xxv US News and World Report (2020) Top Ranked Hospitals for Rehabilitation. Retrieved from https://www.sci-info-pages.com/top-rehabilitation-hospitals/

xxvi ASHA (2014) Telepractice Retrieved from http://www.asha.org/Practice-Portal/Professional-Issues/Telepractice/.

xxvii American Speech-Language-Hearing Association (2020) Medicare Part B Review Process for Therapy Claims. Retrieved from: https://www.asha.org/Practice/reimbursement/medicare/Medicare-Part-B-Review-Process-for-Therapy-Claims/

xxviii Medicare.gov (2020) Speech-Language Pathology Services. Retrieved from: https://www.medicare.gov/coverage/speech-language-pathology-services

xxix Royal College of Speech Language Therapists (2011) Why do people lose friends after a stroke? Retrieved from: http://www.ncbi.nlm.nih.gov/pubmed/21899670

xxx HOPES. (June 26, 2010). HOPES Huntington Outreach Project for Education at Stanford. Retrieved from: http://www.stanford.edu/group/hopes/cgi-bin/wordpress/2010/06/neuroplasticity/

xxxi Perlmutter, David MD,. (November 2, 2010). Neurogenesis: How to Change Your Brain. Retrieved from http://www.huffingtonpost.com/dr-david-perlmutter-md/neurogenesis-what-it-mean_b_777163.html

xxxii Giroux, Holistic Brain Health better living for MS, Parkison's, Dystonia Stroke: Neuroplasticity. retrieved from HYPERLINK

"http://drgiroux.com/neuroplasticity/Holistic"
http://drgiroux.com/neuroplasticity/

Stroke Connection Magazine (September/October 2004)Constraint induced movement therapy retrieved from http://www.strokeassociation.org/STROKEORG/LifeAfterStroke/RegainingIndependence/PhysicalChallenges/Constraint-Induced-Movement-Therapy_UCM_309798_Article.jsp

Giroux, Holistic Brain Health better living for MS, Parkison's, Dystonia Stroke: Neuroplasticity. retrieved from HYPERLINK "http://drgiroux.com/neuroplasticity/Holistic" http://drgiroux.com/neuroplasticity/

[xxxv]ASHA, (2014) Aphasia Treatments. Retrieved from http://www.asha.org/PRPSpecificTopic.aspx?

[xxxvi] Palmer, R., Enderby, P., et al. (2013). Using Computers to Enable Self-Management of Aphasia Therapy Exercises for Word Finding: The Patient and Carer Perspective. Retrieved from http://ncepmaps.org/aphasia/tx/comp-based/

[xxxvii]Friedemann Pulvermüller, PhD,Bettina Neininger, MA,Thomas Elbert, PhD, Bettina Mohr, PhD, Brigitte Rockstroh, PhD. Peter Koebbel, MA, Edward Taub, PhD, (November 11, 2000). **Constraint-Induced Therapy of Chronic Aphasia After Stroke. Retrieved from http://stroke.ahajournals.org/content/32/7/1621.full**

[xxxviii]Helm-Estabrooks, N, Albert, Martin L. (1991). Manual of Aphasia Therapy. Austin Texas: Pro-ed.

[xxxix]Norton, Andrea, Zipse,L, Schlaug, G. (2009) Melodic Intonation Therapy: Shared Insights on How it is Done and Why it Might Help. Retrieved from: http://www.ncbi.nlm.nih.gov/pmc/articles/PMC2780359/

[xl]Helm-Estabrooks, N, Albert, Martin L. (1991). Manual of Aphasia Therapy. Austin Texas: Pro-ed.

[xli]Helm-Estabrooks, N, Albert, Martin L. (1991). Manual of Aphasia Therapy. Austin Texas: Pro-ed.

[xlii]McCaffrey, Patrick. (2008) Neuroscience on the Web Aphasia Therapy. Retrieved from http://www.csuchico.edu/~pmccaffrey/syllabi/SPPA336/336unit10.html

[xliii] Cherney LR, (2010) Oral reading for language in aphasia (ORLA): evaluating the efficacy of computer-delivered therapy in chronic nonfluent aphasia. Retrieved from http://www.ncbi.nlm.nih.gov/pubmed/21239366

[xliv] American Speech-Language-Hearing Association (2020) Retrieved & adapted from: https://www.asha.org/PRPSpecificTopic.aspx?folderid=8589934663§ion=Treatment

[xlv] American Speech-Language-Hearing Association (2020) Retrieved from: https://www.asha.org/PRPSpecificTopic.aspx?folderid=8589934663§ion=Treatment

[xlvi] Simmons-Mackie, N. (2018) Aphasia in North America. Retrieved from: https://www.aphasiaaccess.org/white-papers/

[xlvii]Holland, Audrey, (2011) Developing and Using Scripts in the Treatment of Aphasia. Retrieved from http://www.unm.edu/~atneel/shs531/aphasia-scripts2-handout.pdf

[xlviii] Elsner, B., Kugler, J., et al. (2019).Transcranial Direct Current Stimulation (tDCS) for Improving Aphasia in Adults With Aphasia After Stroke, Retrieved from: https://www.asha.org/ArticleSummary.aspx?id=8589981329

[xlix]ASHA, (2014) Aphasia Treatments. Retrieved from http://www.asha.org/PRPSpecificTopic.aspx?folderid=8589934663§ion=Treatment.

[l]Sutton, M. (2012) App-titude: Apps to Aid Aphasia, ASHA LEADER Retrived from http://www.asha.org/Publications/leader/2012/120605/App-titude—Apps-to-Aid-Aphasia.htm.

[li]Sutton, M. (2012) App-titude: Apps to Aid Aphasia, ASHA LEADER Retrived from http://www.asha.org/Publications/leader/2012/120605/App-titude—Apps-to-Aid-Aphasia.htm.

[lii] Simmons-Mackie, N. (2018) Aphasia in North America. Retrieved from: https://www.aphasiaaccess.org/white-papers/

[liii] Simmons-Mackie, N. (2018) Aphasia in North America. Retrieved from: https://www.aphasiaaccess.org/white-papers/

[liv] Kauhanen ML et al. (2000) Aphasia, depression, and non-verbal cognitive impairment in ischaemic stroke. Retrieved from: http://www.ncbi.nlm.nih.gov/pubmed/11070376

[lv] Kauhanen ML et al. (2000) Aphasia, depression, and non-verbal cognitive impairment in ischaemic stroke. Retrieved from: http://www.ncbi.nlm.nih.gov/pubmed/11070376

[lvi] Jungfer, P, MD. (2014) Depression following Stroke. Retrieved from: http://www.strokensw.org.au/after-a-stroke/depression-following-stroke/

[lvii] Benson, D. and Ardila, A. (1996) Aphasia a Clinical Perspective. Oxford University Press.. Retrieved from: http://books.google.com/books?id=iZ8PfkgGiOUC&pg=PA331&lpg=PA331&dq=aphasia+periods+of+grief&source=bl&ots=UB9h3vrAUm&sig=CpPqDY_hiuTlTp4UOgizzndfVIY&hl=en&sa=X&ei=eRzUU5zaB42yyATt0oL4Cg&ved=0CCgQ6AEwAg#v=onepage&q=aphasia%20periods%20of%20grief&f=false

[lviii] Friedman, R. (2009) No Stages of Grief Retrieved from: HYPERLINK "http://www.psychologytoday.com/blog/broken-hearts/200909/no-stages-grief" http://www.psychologytoday.com/blog/broken-hearts/200909/no-stages-grief

Devine, M. (2013) Stages of Grief and Other Lies that don't help anyone. Retrieved From http://www.huffingtonpost.com/megan-devine/stages-of-grief_b_4414077.html

[lx] National Stroke Foundation (2014) Understanding Emotional Lability. Retrieved from: http://www.strokefoundation.com.au/blog/?tag=emotional-lability

[lxi] National Stroke Foundation (2014) Understanding Emotional Lability. Retrieved from: http://www.strokefoundation.com.au/blog/?tag=emotional-lability

[lxii] Chiu, D. D., & Dow, D. M. (2017). Recovering You Page . In *Healing the Broken Brain* (p. 145). Carlsbad, CA: Hay House, Inc.

[lxiii] National Aphasia Association, (2014) Aphasia Facts Retrieved from http://www.aphasia.org/content/aphasia-faq

[lxiv] Bartels-Tobin, Lori. (2010) Aphasia Survivors Take Charge of Their Own Recovery. Retrieved From: http://www.strokesmart.org/article?id=92.

[lxv] American Stroke Association, (2014) retrieved from: http://powertoendstroke.org/stroke-reduce-risk-controllable.html.

[lxvi] Ira S. Ockene, I,S, MD, & Houston Miller, N. (November 11, 1997).Cigarette Smoking, Cardiovascular Disease, and Stroke A Statement for Healthcare Professionals From the American Heart Association Retrieved from http://circ.ahajournals.org/content/96/9/3243.full

[lxvii] Ira S. Ockene, I,S, MD, & Houston Miller, N. (November 11, 19997).Cigarette Smoking, Cardiovascular Disease, and Stroke A Statement for Healthcare Professionals From the American Heart Association Retrieved from http://circ.ahajournals.org/content/96/9/3243.full

[lxviii] National Stroke Association, (2014) retrieved from: http://www.stroke.org/site/PageServer?pagename=STARS

[lxix] National Stroke Association, (2014) retrieved from: http://www.stroke.org/site/PageServer?pagename=STARS

[lxx] UMN Communication Science department. Retrieved from: HYPERLINK "http://www.d.umn.edu/~mmizuko/2230/sym.htm" http://www.d.umn.edu/~mmizuko/2230/sym.htm

[lxxi] Simmons-Mackie et. al. (2000). Life Participation Approach for Aphasia: A Statement of Values for the future. *ASHA Leader* 5(3):4-6,

Also By David Dow

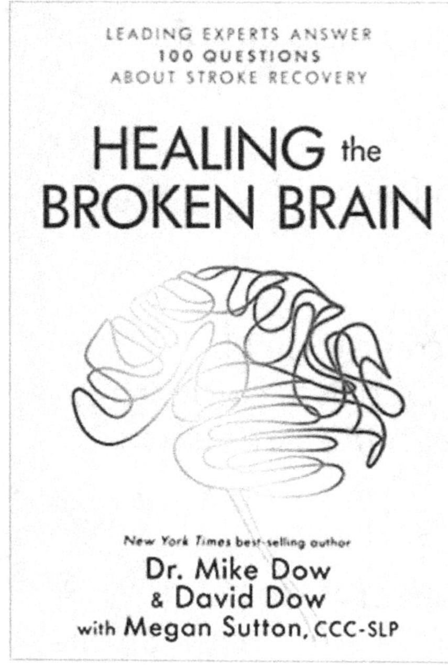

In **Healing the Broken Brain** the top 100 questions about stroke are answered by the top physicians and therapists from around the country. The book is aphasia friendly with takeaway points. Written by David Dow and his brother Dr. Mike Dow with Megan Sutton, CCC-SLP.

Brain Attack shares David's story with frankness, humor, and most of all, with hope. A great motivational read for people coping with aphasia. Click on cover for more information and to order.

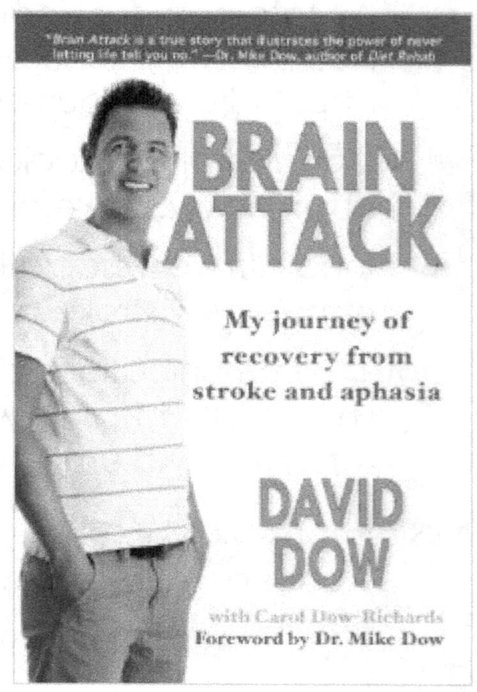

Also by Amanda Anderson MS, CCC, SLP

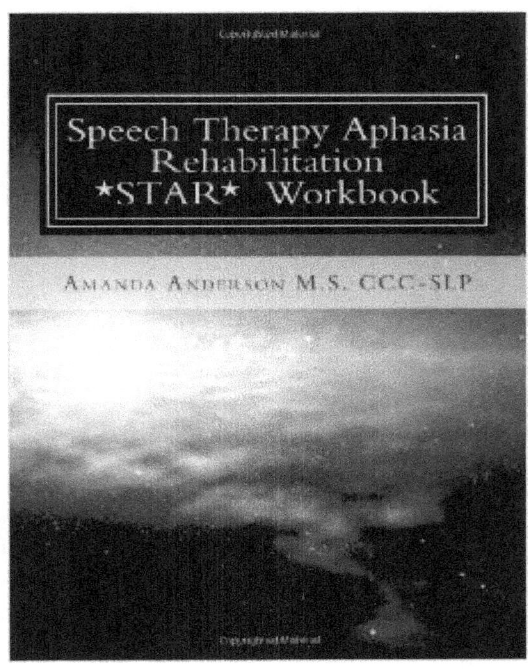

Speech Therapy Aphasia Rehabilitation

**STAR* Workbooks*

A series of three workbooks for people with aphasia to optimize recovery either in therapy or at home. Click on cover to order.

Coming in 2021 from Carol Dow-Richards:
Stroke Warrior